3 STRESS-LESS STEPS TO CONNECT, CLEAR
AND CALM DIGESTION. OWN THE THRONE!

OH, SH*T!

DR. MARISOL TEIJEIRO
NATUROPATHIC DOCTOR
A.K.A THE QUEEN OF THE THRONES™

BALBOA.PRESS
A DIVISION OF HAY HOUSE

Balboa Press books may be ordered through booksellers or by contacting:

Balboa Press
A Division of Hay House
1663 Liberty Drive
Bloomington, IN 47403
www.balboapress.com
1 (877) 407-4847

Because of the dynamic nature of the Internet, any web addresses or links contained in this book may have changed since publication and may no longer be valid. The views expressed in this work are solely those of the author and do not necessarily reflect the views of the publisher, and the publisher hereby disclaims any responsibility for them.

The author of this book does not dispense medical advice or prescribe the use of any technique as a form of treatment for physical, emotional, or medical problems without the advice of a physician, either directly or indirectly. The intent of the author is only to offer information of a general nature to help you in your quest for emotional and spiritual well-being. In the event you use any of the information in this book for yourself, which is your constitutional right, the author and the publisher assume no responsibility for your actions.

Any people depicted in stock imagery provided by Getty Images are models, and such images are being used for illustrative purposes only. Certain stock imagery © Getty Images.

Edited by Victoria Williams, Natalie Glavovic, Brad Luelo, Elke Whitmore

Illustrated by Marielle Graham

Printed in the United States of America.

ISBN: 978-1-9822-4077-6 (sc)
ISBN: 978-1-9822-4078-3 (hc)
ISBN: 978-1-9822-4076-9 (e)

Library of Congress Control Number: 2020900336

Balboa Press rev. date: 05/15/2020

PRAISE FOR OH, SH*T!

"If the poop grosses you out, get over yourself; read the book to understand what your stool is telling you about your digestion - the epicenter of your health. Dr. Marisol does a fantastic job in making poop a relatable, funny and easily digestible topic, with solid action plans how to fix it. A must-read." -Magdalena Wszelaki, Hormone & Nutrition Expert

"Dr. Marisol takes the taboo subject of toilet troubles and delivers the science and solutions for those with IBS. She makes it fun, approachable and totally surmountable! You won't be able to put it down!" -Robyn Openshaw, Bestselling Author

"If you have struggled with digestion, please read Dr. Marisol's book, Oh, Sh*t! Yes, the book is lighthearted and comedic - the title makes me laugh just from typing it - but please know that you'll get more than just entertainment. Dr. Marisol is a naturopathic physician who has made it her mission to help those with the most difficult cases of irritable bowel syndrome regain control over digestive symptoms. I respect her work and highly recommend this book." -Dr. Alan Christianson, Bestselling Author

"Say goodbye to the bloat and an irritable bowel and hello to a beautiful flat belly. Dr. Marisol's book, Oh, Sh*t! is easy to digest and full of royal gems that transform your digestion from stressed to blessed. It's a delicious and inspiring read that will keep you coming back for seconds." -JJ Virgin, New York Times Bestselling Author of The Virgin Diet

To my mother, my guiding lights, my angel, my 22.
To the woman that gave me all of her, including her light.
Mama cuando me diste Luz, me diste el mundo.
You continue to live through me, I am
your legacy. I wrote this for you.
I will forever remember your hugs, your
kisses, your tucking-me-in at night.
I will always honour your kindness, generosity, love,
genius, passion for learning, languages, music and dance
and dedication to making things better for all.
I will travel with you always in my heart.
You will always be by my side.
Love you Mamá, Para siempre.

CONTENTS

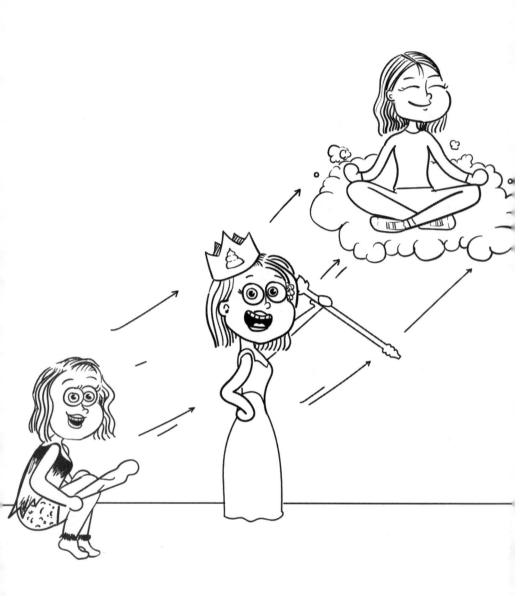

OH, SH*T!

Oh, Sh*t! Every time I hear myself or someone else say this I chuckle. Why? Not because I have a trucker mouth, but more because it's incredible how the human existence operates. Our vocabulary and phrases are created based on our experience, and it's no shocker that humans have been dealing with sh*t for quite a long time.

Oh Sh*t! Isn't just a simple saying, but a deep insight into the life of those dealing with irritable bowel syndrome (IBS), inflammatory bowel disease like Crohn's or colitis, constipation and any other chronic disease such as cancer, autoimmune, or hormone problems where you can't poo. Oh Sh*t! Is that feeling you get when you don't know where the next toilet is and you are about to have an accident. The anxiety you feel going somewhere new and not knowing whether they will have toilets. The feeling you feel when you haven't gone to the bathroom in a few days. Oh, Sh*t! Where the heck is it? Will it ever come out?!

Yes it will! This book contains the recipe to achieve that miracle time and time again. Even more, this book will help you to achieve great digestion each and every time you chew. Digestion should be that place where food and you meet on a harmonious plane; where what you eat makes you feel fabulous. There are no ifs, ands or butts about it! (Pun intended). It's that place where you always have a flat stomach (yes, this is possible) and you don't need to take a nap after your meal. You feel energized by what you have eaten and you're not always hungry for more.

When people are describing their digestion, they refer to their guts, their bowel, their intestines, their stomach and many other random names that people decide to use… sometimes I have no idea what they are even talking about. I've realized, over time, that all these names make it confusing for my patients. So, I decided to simplify and to give the digestive place a special name that would refer to the processes that are happening with all of the digestive organs, whatever you choose to call them. I call it the "D-Spot". You will read it throughout this book as I will help you to connect and find your D-Spot, just like I have found mine. The 'D-Spot' is much more sexy than 'digestion', don't you think?

So how did I find my D-Spot? Well, it hasn't been all that easy and it has taken me quite some time. I was fortunate to be in the right place and open to receiving possibilities at the right time. I had, in essence, been prepared enough and explored enough and I'm sure no different than you, began to notice the signs and synchronicities placed in my way by the universe. My yellow brick road began to unfold on my journey to healing. For me, it began first with a friend and then with a book and then with a job. The book that changed my life was a cult classic in natural medicine, found in the recesses of most health food stores, written by a naturopathic doctor. The job took me on a learning journey where I gained so much expertise in cleansing medicine and taught naturopathic doctors how to cleanse and heal their patients. I had no choice but to become a naturopathic doctor and as it turned out, I was a natural at natural medicine!

The biggest blessing was that of being in enough pain to realize that I personally needed to change, and everything that I was learning was meant to heal me, not only with the knowledge but with the actual implementation of tools and techniques. You too can touch your D-Spot. Your journey is laid out for you in this book but only if you're willing to play along and do the work it takes to get you there. We can do this together.

The journey laid out for you in this book has been formulated from my experience. I've tried most every treatment and all the hippie healing stuff I could get my hands on. Some I've loved and others I've lost, they just didn't resonate with me. I've probably read close to 85% of the health books that are out there and like you, I'm a true health seeker. I've Dr. Googled more than the average and given myself a few interesting, yet not real diagnoses.

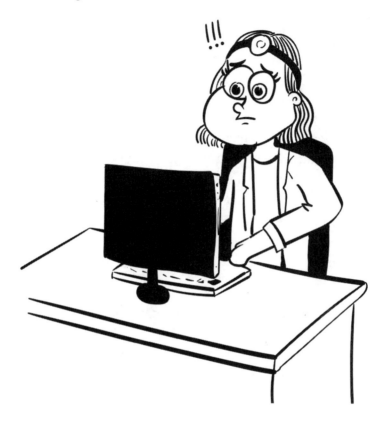

I want to know what is going on and I just can't get enough. What I learn, I experience, and then I teach. For me, as a naturopathic doctor, teaching helps me to learn it better. Even before I was a naturopathic doctor I was trying to teach it to whomever would listen, because I really wanted to master the information so that my body would follow. I encourage you to do the same through this book; teach your friends so that YOU can really practise what you are teaching. Some of you may not be there yet, and some people may not be willing to listen, but that is okay. Teach anyway! This will help to make all the jewels of this book completely natural to you; part of who you are, engrained in your neural networks, like they are in mine after years of practice and practise.

What you are about to embark on is my inner exploration over the past 15 years to improve my health. I was diagnosed with asthma as a kid, that was actually severe anxiety. I lived at that time, chronically constipated, dealing with the addiction of smoking and overeating the wrong type of foods. I've been heavy and I've been too skinny. I had polycystic ovarian syndrome (PCOS), which almost stopped me from going to school because I was so worried that I wouldn't be able to have kids if I didn't fix myself first. Further, I had mononucleosis and was forced to take a semester off of school. Later I dealt with irritable bowel syndrome (IBS), a resurgence of my anxiety as a child, but in a different form. My experiences, in turn, helped frame my operandus clinicus (fancy, make-believe half latin word for the way I roll) in my naturopathic clinic at Sanas Health Practice. My team and I have helped thousands of patients from all over the world. This book is to continue that trend and to help you where you are at right now. You may not be able to come up to visit us, but this book is like we are at home with you, WELCOME!

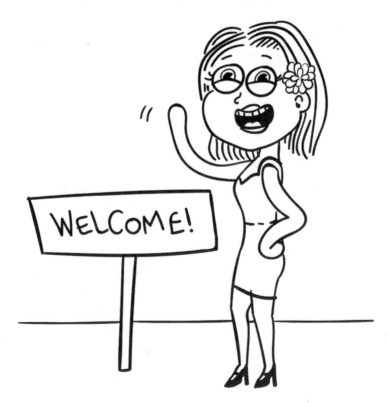

My focus has been to create a safe haven, a place for those who need to clear the pain and step into their lives. One hundred percent of our treatments begin with regulating digestion. Why? Because digestion is where life begins. If you are to reclaim your life from the outside, you must first begin with your insides. That was the biggest lesson in my life, and what I will teach you here. **Every movement, literally, begins from within. Let's start your movement now.**

What motivates and moves me, you, us to change? It's simple - pain. Pain is one of life's greatest motivators and it is through pain that we are able to best evolve. Change evolves through pain. Think about it like this - when you are physically injured you are unable to move the way you are accustomed. Pain forces you to adapt to the situation, to modify your behaviours, to switch it up, so you can achieve the best quality of life for yourself, here and now.

Many people consider pain to be the reason we refuse to change, but in reality, it is the guiding force of our evolution. Pain is our gift. It is the symptom in our lives telling us that we are not in the right place. It's a gift with a double edged sword. On one side, it causes you such enormous pressure, unrest and irritation, leaving you unhappy and disconnected. On the other side, it creates that internal fire that forges the way ahead, creating the pathway to our divine expression and the realization of our spirit.

You could always choose to simply numb the pain, using a multitude of substances, medical drugs and distractions, like a pain reliever or an aspirin. Or how about an antidepressant or anti-anxiety medicine to relieve symptoms; these are the drugs of choice for those suffering with irritable bowels. Why not? That is a choice. I have said yes to that choice on multiple occasions, I've been no angel. I've abused my temple and my beautiful body. I understand the pain of food cravings, sometimes you just can't help yourself. I feel for those who want to quit smoking. I've been there, done that. I've lived in those shoes and through living it, I know you can get through it as I did. But the only way out, is through it. Unfortunately (or fortunately), there is no by-pass. You can't suppress the pain and expect to get better for real.

The reality is at the end of the day, if you choose to numb your pain without addressing the root cause, the pain won't really go away. When you go into your bed to rest, rest comes not. Your pain will be multiplied internally in the still of the night, in your place of rest you will be stressed. The upheaval will come from within, your self will tell you what you need. It will bring you the clarity that you need for life. You just need to listen, go into the pain and grow.

I don't regret those times, or any of my choices, and when it happens, or the pattern repeats, just remember life is a journey. I look at it as a blessing and a time to reset. My having experienced this pain and to have experienced the numbing, is allowing me to know yours. We are the same, we are having similar experiences and knowing that, allows me to better help you.

You picking up this book is your way of saying to the universe, *"I'm done, I'm ready to change."*

So let's say it here and now, out loud and proud. **Oh, Sh*t!** Notice what it feels like to say this, how it resonates with all the emotions, feelings and sensations you have been living with. From here on in this saying will take on a whole new meaning to you as will your life.

CHAPTER 1

TOUCH YOUR D-SPOT

Your D-Spot (A.K.A. the digestive spot) is the most intimate part of your body. It's the part of you that connects you to you. When I discovered this, it made a lot of sense. In my life I was doing patchwork for my health and never really feeling awesome, never feeling really good inside. When I began to focus on my D-Spot, it improved my entire life, like it will for you.

It is the deepest innermost part of your body. It is the outside world on the inside of your body. Only two plus a few trillion know what it feels like... you, food and the trillions of bugs that share your D-Spot. Boy, you are promiscuous! Unfortunately, the food you eat isn't able to comment on how great or unhappy your D-Spot is, because it loses itself within you, becoming modified along the way. But the bugs that live within your gut certainly do make some noise, and you hear from them in a multitude of ways. Passing bad gas and floating poops are just to name a few examples. Oh, Sh*t!

Only you can work to achieve a divine D-Spot and live to comment about it. When you have a dynamic, divine D-Spot, it's like heaven. You are on top of the world and nothing compares to it, except maybe an earth-shattering orgasm. You are intuitively connected to the universe and connected to how you feel. There are no blockages from bloating, constipation, diarrhea or cravings. Wouldn't it be great to have a mind blowing D-Spot and consistent earth shattering orgasms? Well I say, why not? Life is meant to be lived and lived fabulously. Life is how you digest and it simply takes guts to go deep inside.

The D-Spot is the most important part of your body and digestion is the most important function of the body. Without proper digestion, it is impossible to create health. The food that comes in must be processed properly, absorbed through a healthy and integral gut lining with good bacteria, and then nutrients are utilized to support metabolism, the immune system, hormones, neurotransmitters and a healthy brain. The waste products must come out regularly as well.

If you imagine it, our digestive tract is one great big tube. It has an opening on one end, your mouth, and an opening on the other, your anus. Food and drink comes in one way and out the other. Mid-way, there has to be a processing plant for us to utilize what we need to survive. This tube (the entire length of the D-Spot) is the outside world on our insides.

There are trillions of inhabitants in our D-Spots. Hopefully, they are beneficial bacteria and some yeasts, but not disease-causing ones. Let's call them bugs, because that's basically what they are. These bugs help to process nutrients. If they are the right type of healthy bugs, they are essential to help us improve our health and immunity. Unhealthy bugs are detrimental to our D-Spot and disrupt our ability to find balance in our health[1].

An unhealthy, damaged D-Spot is where physiological, emotional and toxic stress contribute to unhealthy bugs and gaps, referenced by some as leaky guts[2]. In our D- spot, this causes a variety of physiological responses. Most importantly, chronic inflammation[3], the root of all disease that can severely damage your D-Spot, causing you to lose the delight you once had in your life.

Irritable bowel syndrome (IBS) is a condition involving a damaged D-Spot that presents as pain, bloating, distension and difficult bowel habits. There is often a predominance or alternation of diarrhea and constipation. It affects 10-20% of the western world. Those who suffer often report a strong psychological association with anxiety and stress[4].

To diagnose, it is often done by exclusion, meaning there isn't a true test to conclude that you have it, although there are some in the works[5]. Most sufferers go through a gamut of tests to rule out inflammatory bowel disease such as Crohn's disease or ulcerative colitis and other more ominous conditions such as gastrointestinal cancer. There are certain commonalities found in irritable bowel syndrome patients. As an example, more often than not, small intestine bacterial overgrowth (SIBO) is present. It's a condition that is debilitating for many and majorly impacts quality of life. This is why people who deal with this on a regular basis, as I did, desperately need to balance their D-Spot.

Beyond the physical effects of balancing the D-Spot, tuning into your D-Spot makes you more connected to the universe, God, the one, or whatever you choose to call it. I remember the clarity of mind that came with improving my D-Spot; that was my first sign. Tough life decisions become easier to make because you are more connected to your needs. It's a constant work in progress but the payback is huge. When you treat your D-Spot divinely, it will connect you to the divine.

The D-Spot is also intimately connected to your brain, your emotions[6] and most importantly, your intuition. In fact, the digestive tract is known as the second brain and in my opinion, your connection to the universe. Think of butterflies in your belly; if you are in tune with your body, you can feel multiple emotions in your belly. You have a sick feeling in your stomach when something just doesn't feel right. Neurotransmitters, that are messengers of the nervous system like serotonin[7] [8] and GABA[9], for example, are found in high concentrations in a healthy D-Spot.

To have a healthy D-Spot you must have a good balance of these neurotransmitters, hormones and immune system function[10]. But the reverse is also true. You can't create healthy messengers for the body if you're unable to nourish yourself properly.

Did you know many of the sufferers of an imbalanced D-Spot have coexisting anxiety problems[11]? Anxiety plays a huge role in the health of your D-Spot. The D-Spot can also respond to hormones, immune system messengers and chemicals expressed from the bacteria, yeast and the food present in the D-Spot.

Your mission, should you choose to accept it, is to create your own personal divine D-Spot. Life is about creation, and creation is truly joyous. Having an incredibly healthy digestive tract allows you to experience your own personal bliss, and you will be able to deal with everything life throws at you with grace and clarity.

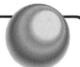

PEARL OF WISDOM

Did you know that your D-Spot is the only area of your body that has its very own nervous system, its own 'brain'? It's called the enteric nervous system, or The Second Brain[12], according to Dr. Gershon. How good you feel in your digestive tract can influence the way your whole body feels. That's one of the reasons it's so important to take good care of your D-Spot so that you feel great!

Food Refresh

In our society food has become a major pastime. People spend hours focused on it, obsessing over it; breaking it down to each of its finer parts; calories, protein, carbohydrates, fats and micronutrients. They take the whole out of the wheat, the lactose out of the milk, they overcook, over process, and worst of all, they over consume.

Food used to be a necessity to survive, since it was scarce. With the overabundance of commercial food creation, we have so much, that we intend to eat it all. Obesity is at an all-time high, not only in adults, but sadly, in children as well. Our diet is referred to as the Standard American Diet, A.K.A. SAD. It is full of over-processed, fast convenience food that is deplete of true nourishment. I don't know if that acronym was created on purpose but it pretty much sums it all up. Many of our diets truly are SAD at this point.

I grew up with a diet that by many standards was considered perfect, not SAD. Whole foods came from our garden and everything was made from scratch. It's funny how you and your perspective changes. I was so wishing that my dad would buy packaged and processed foods, because that's what all the other kids ate and I didn't want to be so different, bringing sardine sandwiches to school.

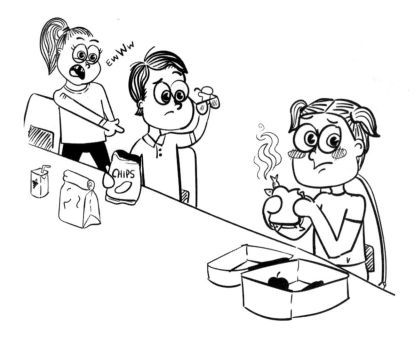

Since we were poor, everything was made from scratch to stretch the dollar, which was a problem but also a Godsend. The only thing was, what stretched the dollar was typically a meal very heavy in carbohydrates and starches. Potatoes and rice on a plate were a common occurrence. There was little protein to be seen at my house. My mother would always complain, *"Where's the beef?"*, citing a popular commercial from the 80's. In fact, it was the running joke at our house. We were setting ourselves up to become carbohydrate addicts, trained to eat large quantities of carbs to fill the void of other nutrients. Carbohydrates, whether they come in the form of starches, fruits, legumes or vegetables, vary in their glucose content. Some affect your blood glucose levels more than others, but all act as sugar, as they eventually break down into sugars.

For many, carbohydrates don't fill you up. It's proteins and fats that turn off the switch to continue eating. We ate a lot and had an abundance of good quality food, but the amount, as well as the composition of our plates, left much to be desired from a health perspective. We were feeding our addiction to carbohydrates and stressing our bodies because we were depleted in nutrients and proteins. This caused an uproar in our bodies and depleted our serotonin levels.

Lack of protein can cause a deficiency in neurotransmitters such as serotonin, dopamine and GABA. We can't make these happy messengers without the raw materials. Protein is necessary. Ironically, a deficiency in the body of these feel good substances will leave you craving carbohydrates which will momentarily make up for the lack. It's just a temporary fix and you keep on feeling deficient until you fuel up on the raw material to make it. We need protein in our diet, carbohydrates alone are not the solution. This is why I believe in the ancestral paleo diet, and fasting for health. It just makes sense, and the D-Spot Meal Practice that you will learn about in this book is based upon these principles.

What's really interesting is with all this abundance, you would think we would be happier and more satiated! The problem is, we were not consuming the right combination of food, as my example showed, and the opposite is true. Unsatisfied with life, people run to their doctors and get anti-depressant prescriptions to ease their personal dissatisfaction. Depression and mood-based disorders are all on the rise, likely because a component of all of these is nutrient deficiencies, and when food is void of essential nutrients, the brains (both the one in your head and the one in your D-Spot - no, not in your pants) don't function appropriately. So you don't feel good and you lack satisfaction in what you eat, and in your life. So guess what? You keep on trying to fill that void to survive.

We are better fed, but hungrier. How does this make sense? The perfect example is diabetes. Did you know in alternative medical circles, it's described as "starvation in a land of plenty"? Type II diabetes, the one that is typically caused by diet, can be reversed. It is when there are ample amounts of sugar, and it doesn't necessarily need to be from candy, soft drinks or fast food, contrary to popular belief[13]. In fact, over feeding and having too many snacks overwhelms the body with sugar (glucose, the molecule that allows us to grow). However, there is so much of it, that the body says, "Whoa... no more of this, thank you" so the cells stop absorbing it. The sugar floats around aimlessly, waging a war in our blood and on our tissues, including the nervous system. This explains the heart disease, neuropathies and decline in eyesight that are all classical sequelae of dealing with this chronic disease. It's hard to believe that something as innocent as sugar can be such a trouble maker. Remember my family? Our diets resulted in my having insulin resistance and PCOS at a very young age and my parents being diagnosed with Type II diabetes at a later date. All conditions are ruled and regulated by excess sugar in the diet and an inability to regulate between carbohydrate and fat metabolism[14]. That which gives life can also take it away. The basic conundrum here is there is too much of a good thing and the body loses the ability to properly respond to it.

Food is more than just the sum of its parts. It's not something that you can compartmentalize. Food is a method of communication with our body, what is called a biological response modifier[15], which means it actually acts very similar to a hormone, neurotransmitter or other biochemical messenger, commanding and instructing the body to function in certain ways. Food isn't merely for taste, it is much more powerful than that. Every morsel that passes your lips commands your entire mind, body and soul to function in a specific way. There is no denying it. Food is extremely powerful! It can heal the body, it can cause stress and anxiety to the body or it can control the body by creating a dependency.

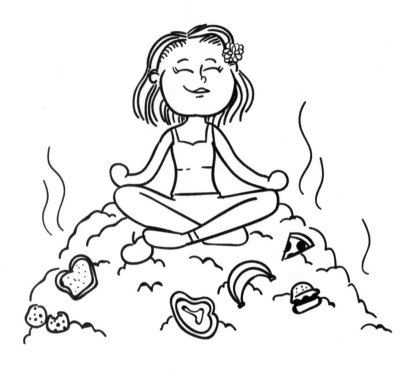

Food addiction was once a beneficial evolutionary tool, an instinct. It embedded into our DNA due to the scarcity of food in our palaeolithic ancestors' diet, the hunters and gatherers[16]. The main issue nowadays is with the over-processed high sugar, high fat and high salt content of our food supply. Our bodies are overstimulated, and readjusting to the new levels of stimulation which have perpetuated our being in an ongoing binge. We can't get enough. Of course, when something you intake makes you feel good, why wouldn't you seek that out?

The most genetically engraved addiction is the taste for sugar, or rather the effect that sugar has on our bodies. If you break it down to the basic physiology, all addictive substances have a similar cascade of effects on the body and an effect on the nervous system, stimulating the dopamine reward centers[17], making you feel temporarily euphoric. There is also an effect on all other regulatory systems in the body, specifically the immune system via the glucocorticoid pathway. This pathway interconnects all the systems and organs and is how the body either "promotes or prevents adaptation to stress"[18]. The interesting thing is that the glucocorticoid molecule is very similar to the sugar molecule. Sugar naturally stresses the system; that stress can make you feel good. The focus is always all on the food, but truth is, we are searching to stimulate this system in a certain way, no matter the substance.

Take alcohol, which is in effect, liquid sugar. When you look at the label you will see it is extremely high in calories and carbohydrates. Because it's sugar, it will stimulate the stress systems and on top of that it gives you a loopy feeling due to the fermentation by-products being neurotoxic! The numb feeling that comes with drinking greater amounts of alcohol just enhances the addiction potential, as well as the dangerousness of the substance.

What about foods like wheat and dairy? These are also highly addictive and should be used with caution. Interestingly enough, they are both a form of sugar from the carbohydrates in bread (glucose) and milk (lactose). To sweeten the pot, so to say, these substances have an opiate-like effect when consumed and digested[19] [20] [21]. Certain peptides, namely gluten and casein, stimulate the opiate pathway in our bodies. So now, not only do you love them because they taste so good, but you also get the extra bonus of an opiate kick. No kidding that these foods have become such staples in our cultivating farmers' society.

In the past, our addiction to sugar was purposeful. For the paleolithic hunters and gatherers, this meant they would fill up on fruits (when available), usually ripest right before winter, so that they could put on a layer of fat to survive the long winter months inside a cave. For the farmers of the cultivating era, this meant grain silos and keeping cattle warm in the winter inside of barns to supply the liquid gold and preserve the fat supply when fresh food wouldn't be available. Now in our world of overabundance, this can be dangerous in more ways than one. Sugar, in all its forms, from simple to complex carbohydrate, is by far the most epidemic of addictions. Ironically, it is from something that helps us grow and gives us life. That which gives us life can also take it away. How can this be?

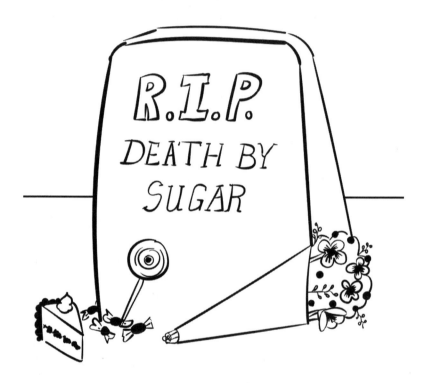

The Irony of Life -- Too Much of a Good Thing, How Can That Be Bad?

The saying is true that too much of a good thing can be detrimental to our health. Everything is about dosage. As a naturopathic doctor, I'm all too familiar with this principle. All poison in the right amount can actually become medicine. Believe it or not, I work on this principle regularly, and all medicine in the wrong amount can become poison.

Consider this, a simple aspirin in the right dose functions as a pain reliever and treats inflammation and fever. Take too much of it, and it can shut your liver function down and kill you. One of my teachers always used to tell me, it's all in the dose. A little sun does the body great! Too much sun and you get a sunburn.

This is the dichotomy of life, or the yin and yang of life. The very best example is sugar, that which helps us grow and thrive. But consider this, a recent study showed that higher than normal blood sugar actually physically shrunk a part of the brain[22a]! This is mind blowing, or actually mind crunching!

Side note: Yin and yang - a principle of taoist philosophy that is an essential element of life and governs all that is. Yin and Yang are opposite forces, interconnected, mutually creating, interdependent in the natural world. Yang is light, bright, male energy while yin is heavy, dark, female energy. One can't exist without the other. If there is no darkness, there can be no light. Opposites are required to give rise to each other. What is good can make bad. Without the ebb, there is no flow, without sad there can be no happy.

The problem is complicated because higher blood glucose is associated with higher levels of the stress hormone, cortisol, in the body[22b]. Stress causes our body to liberate and increase our natural reserves of blood sugar and insulin so that sugar can go into the cells instead of floating about, wreaking havoc. So if you're eating sugar all of the time, yes, you will achieve the high on life and the fast and fleeting feel-good sensation that sugar brings you, which ironically, is how you feel when under stress. The only difference is how you perceive it. Obviously, the milkshake you are enjoying goes down much better than the fact that you may be staring down a lion's throat. The big problem is that longterm stress and elevation of blood sugar leads to insulin resistance[23]. This sets you up for metabolic syndrome and consequently, diabetes.

This pattern is mimicked time and again, purposefully. Sugar for our body becomes a dangerous messenger, telling the body that it is stressed and that it needs to pump out insulin because we need to get all of this sugar into the cells. That's one of the reasons when you're feeling tired, you go for sugar to perk you up instantly. It literally stresses out the body. It's the cascade of physiological effects that your body understands, its morse code. This is similar to the coffee or caffeine perk up which stresses your body to make you feel alert. Too much of these good things can really damage your system. Whether you perceive them as good or bad, the body knows its signals.

The other facet of this is that if you need, crave or want too much of one thing, are you not possibly addicted to it? You likely are, and with addiction comes dependence and loss of freedom. A weakening of your entire being. You lose your will. You lose the things that are important to you. You lose **you**. You become possessed to act, think, breathe, eat, and live by the substance that owns you, that holds you in its grasp. The substance has basically caged you. You are a slave. You're overtaken, moment by moment; all of your thoughts go to that substance and when you can get it next, so you can feel again, and again, and again, like you do when you're on it. You know it's not good for you, yet you can't help yourself. You know better. Why then, can't you do better?

How do we get so entangled into these simple addictions like sugar and food, basic substances necessary for life? It's as nature intended. First we like it, then we learn how to get it and then internally we want it really badly[24]. What happens over time is that we like the reward we get out of it so much that we simply forget to realign. We keep on searching and searching and searching until we get the high.

Are you so low, lacking willpower, losing your own integrity? Are you so ill-willed that you cannot get through this? This is not the case. It's not that you don't have any willpower. It's simply that you haven't chosen differently. You haven't chosen to put the brakes on. You haven't yet chosen to do anything in your power to create the environment suitable for your change. The thing is this: restriction won't "cure" addiction. Only **you** can choose to change your behaviour. You have to want it. For lack of better words, you need to be hungry, really hungry for change.

Now is your time, as the Latin slogan for the United Farm Workers still rings in the ears of the latino population, "SI SE PUEDE". Or as Obama in his 2008 presidential campaign put it, "Yes we can!". It's time! Let this book be your instigator and stimulant for change. My intent is to make you hungry for the change that you need for you to achieve your divine D-Spot.

Together we can unleash our inner movement. Ready, set, roll up those sleeves like Rosie the Riveter… Let's digest. DIG IN!

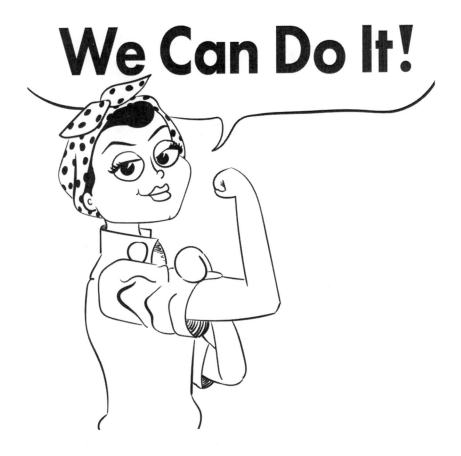

CHAPTER 2

THE ADDICTION WITHIN

I have an addictive personality, and I know I'm not alone. I've struggled through my life with strong addictions to sugar, cigarettes and coffee. They owned me and they ruled my every thought. They commanded my life. It was hard to learn to honour these addictions, and it took me just about until I hit rock bottom, just like everyone says, that I learned to live with them. For me, it wasn't only being addicted to something that was the problem, but the substances that I was choosing were actually part and parcel of the problem. Caffeine and nicotine stimulate the nervous system and I'm an easily excited person with a predisposition to anxiety. Oh, Sh*t!!! These substances served their purpose to make me feel normal, which for me at the time was being in an anxious state. But they also affected my D-Spot negatively. They made me poop like a champ. At the time, I thought it was a godsend, coming from a history of having constipation. But these little too loosey-goosey poopies were because my D-Spot was being irritated by my addictions.

Starting my day with stimulants was the worst thing that I could be doing. These two drugs of choice, nicotine and caffeine, would initially make me feel great and alert but would amp up my anxiety. It became so bad that I started having insomnia, I would stay up all night. Then severe panic attacks of the variety where I thought I was literally dying. It was so horrible. I remember one time curling up into a little ball on the floor as I was hyperventilating with my arms and hands all in spasms. I was completely freaking out. If you've ever experienced a panic attack, you know how life altering the experience can be and that you would do anything to prevent it. This experience was a gift, although initially I didn't see it like that.

Beyond the addictions, there was a part of me that felt so out of tune. I was severely wrestling with myself and my integrity as a person. This wasn't who I wanted to be. Here I was in school in my third year of naturopathic medicine, closet smoking on my balcony. What a hypocrite I was being! I knew I needed a way out, but it was really hard to see that way out because I was self medicating to deal with all of my stress.

I smoked and drank coffee before I showered in the morning and after I returned from school. It kept me from socializing and going out to events with friends because once I had a cigarette, I smelt like it and I didn't want to be labeled a fraud. The only issue was that you can run from others' judgement, but it's pretty hard to run from what you think of yourself. I couldn't keep on running; there was nowhere to hide.

The fact was that school was tough, super stressful and demanding, as it made us look inward for our reasons for wanting to become naturopathic doctors. It challenged our will and stamina everyday. Did I really want to be slaving away like this in school? Did I really want to get so close to patients only to have them leave this world, un-love me or simply disappear, never to be heard from again? You invest so much time in them. Did I really want to learn how delicate health is and how it could be gone in a second? Naturopathic school meant deeply reflecting and examining all of my emotions, my intuition, and instincts, which I learned were all connected deeply to my D-Spot.

My D-Spot Speaks My Mind

You must be thinking, "What does anxiety and addiction have to do with finding my D-Spot?" The truth is, they are intimately connected. First of all, many of our habits and addictions are negatively affecting our D-Spots. Think of sugar addictions, food addictions, cigarette smoking and alcohol consumption, guilty! Oh, Sh*t!!

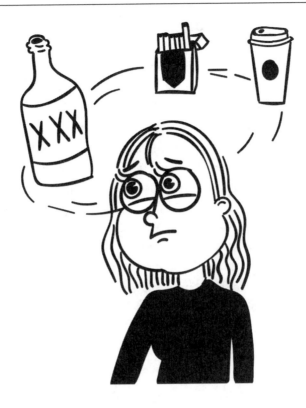

Secondly, our D-Spots are affected by strong overwhelming emotions, like anxiety, because they create stress. I'm sure you've heard of people, that when stressed, keep running to the bathroom[25]. I'm one of those sufferers and let me tell you, when you make the mind-body connection, it's significantly easier to manage and work through. My D-Spot speaks my mind and is a reflection of my inner state of being. Yours feels you too. If I'm not voicing my needs, my concerns or my worries; my D-Spot will surely do a fine job of bringing it up to the surface for me.

Stress hormones keep our digestive tract in an unregulated place and this can be seen in the elite athletes that suffer from D-Spot drama[26] like diarrhea and irritable bowel-like symptoms. You can run but you simply cannot hide. Your D-Spot cannot achieve balance until you give yourself a break. A major part of the treatment plan in this book is to assess, reduce and remove the physical stress on your body, which is creating a repeating cycle of anxiety, stress and addiction.

Addiction and Anxiety Infinity Loop

Addiction and anxiety co-exist and co-create with each other - I like to refer to them as the two peas in the infinity loop pod. We don't know which came first. Was it anxiety and then the addiction? Or does the addiction bring on the anxiety? Often times you are addicted to those things that make you increasingly anxious. And those things that you are addicted to will deplete your nutrient profile, so that your anxiety gets worse. It's a vicious cycle and a lose, lose situation.

What we do know is that they always go hand in hand[27], there is a psychopathology associated with abuse and addictive disorders. The remarkable thing is that both have the ability to evolve us into something greater than we are today. There are gifts within these chains, if we choose to accept them.

Anxiety

You, like me, like most, have felt the terror of anxiety. That overwhelming sensation of pressure on your chest, your heart beating from within, exploding out of your body. You feel it difficult to take a deep breath, a tingling numbing sensation in your hand, mouth, chest, and wherever you have pain. You have pressure in the back of your neck that does not cease, no matter how much you roll your head. Everyone tells you to breathe, but you simply cannot do it. You feel oxygen deficient, like the air around you is empty and you can't get any nourishment from it.

If you have ever been anxious or have felt the feeling of being unable to control the sensations in your body, as those with irritable bowel syndrome do, you know anxiety. The ultimate sensation and lasting feeling is that of not being safe. Feeling a total loss of control. You feel as though at any moment, you could lose everything, everything you have ever worked for. You could lose your whole life! Anxiety makes you feel as though you have lost complete control of your world. So do irritable bowels. Oh, Sh*t!

Anxiety is ultimately inhibiting. It can stop you completely in your tracks. It also extends far beyond your mental state as it can stop or over activate your D-Spot completely. Maybe you are one of those persons, who, when anxious, simply loses your appetite and cannot eat. Others will overeat when anxious to calm the butterflies in their bellies. Some experience an inability to have a good bowel movement and to let go. Still others experience non-stop loose stools. The bottom line is, anxiety can control your life, it can overtake your body, mind and your D-Spot. Time to take back your life.

Why is your D-Spot so emotional? It is simply because it's our outside on the inside. It's innervated by parasympathetic ganglia which are the nervous systems' commanders of the silent, quiet state; the state of rest and digest. Because the D-Spot is so highly innervated, similar to the skin, it's sensation is unique. We still don't have a complete understanding of how intricate the D-Spot is. Research is ongoing as discussed in The Second Brain, by Dr. Michael Gershon. We know it is special!

The sensation of anxiety, as with all things that are uncomfortable, comes bearing a gift. In essence, it's stress, taken up a notch, and it finds its roots in future thinking. You lose control over what will happen in the future, where gloom and doom is the predominant theme. Those that have a tendency towards anxiety, like myself, have the gift of being incredibly **intuitive**. We can feel when things are not right around us. We know when there is unrest. We have this uncanny ability to feel where others cannot. What we choose to do with these feelings is what will either elevate or crush us.

The D-Spot is the vehicle which can feel our intuition. Intuition is important as it guides us to our higher selves. It guides us to a state of lessening stress, of balance and of being in flow. How does it guide us? It guides us through our emotions and sensations, A.K.A. "gut feelings". It may be a nervous feeling that comes with a new decision. It may be a strong confidence when we make a choice that "feels" right. You intimately know when it feels right or wrong; you can feel it in your gut, in your D-Spot. The difference is whether you decide to go forward with the choice that feels right. Do you listen? Do you suppress it with stress or by numbing your feelings? Do you take quiet time to really listen to your intuition or do you simply keep on "doing" and not "being"?

The way towards your intuition is through quiet reflection, meditative practices, castor oil packs, and overall calming down the amount of high energy anxiety or things that may be promoting that in your life. Working on your D-Spot connects you to your intuition and helps you get in touch with your higher self. Over time you become truly in tune with your needs. Your intuition can be curated and cultivated from your anxiety. It is truly a diamond in the rough!

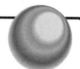

PEARL OF WISDOM

ARE ANXIETY & STRESS THE SAME THING?

Anxiety takes stress to a different level. Stress is constant. There is good stress & bad stress, whereas anxiety is a heightened level of sensation, of impending doom in the upcoming future. The increase in emotion that is seen within anxiety is what opens the doorway towards your intuition.

Addiction

When we talk about addiction in general, it is assumed that the discussion is surrounding a chemical or substance addiction like cigarettes, alcohol or drugs. The reality is that addiction has three faces according to the Diagnostic and Statistical Manual of Mental Disorders (DSM-IV). What is intriguing is that all of the faces of addiction could truly be considered under the umbrella of a substance addiction because the neurobiological effect and the neurotransmitter pathways that are stimulated within our bodies, are all the same. Even so incredible, is that one type of addiction will respond to the treatment used for another type of addiction, such as opioid medications and glutamate modulating substances[28], two key neurotransmitters involved in addiction.

Beyond substances as mentioned above, the second category is food. The search for high calorie and low nutrient foods with a taste for sugar, salt and fat are programmed into our brains as an evolutionary advantage. Feed, so as not to famine[29].

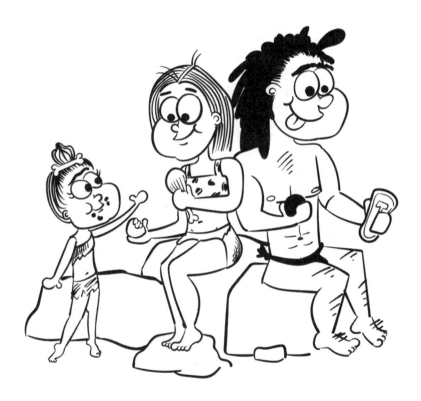

Now we don't need the calories but the food engineers keep on working to improve their foods by making them as addictive as possible. Think about it. Have you ever heard yourself say, "I can't open the package because I will eat it all"? Take chocolate as an example. It contains sugar and fat from the cocoa bean and psychoactive substances, all combined together. It's a recipe for addiction and wanting more[30]. Food addiction is rampant and you are not alone. We are in this one together.

Substance Addiction	Food Addiction	Behavioral Addiction
• Caffeine • Alcohol • Cigarettes • Illegal Drugs	• Sugar • Salt • Fat	• Exercise • Screen Time • Gambling • Sex

The final classification is behavioural addiction. This form extends into exercise, internet addiction, gambling, work, sex and more. Behavioural addiction should not be confused with impulse disorders such as frequently washing hands and checking behaviours[31]. With addiction, the difference is that there is always a tolerance and withdrawal scenario.

According to Freimuth et al, tolerance is where the addict keeps on increasing the substance, food or behaviour to receive the desired effect that will give them their "high". Withdrawal is where, with the lack of their addiction, they begin to desire it more and more and become obsessed with the thought of procuring it. They need their fix. This brings on the feelings of irritability, restlessness, sleeplessness and anxiety[32].

This is why anxiety and addiction are so linked together in the infinity loop. The addiction produces the anxiety. My thoughts are that another unknown part of your affliction may actually be an addiction to the state of being anxious. I know for me, that was my "natural" state, what I would have in the past considered my homeostasis (state of internal balance) as I grew up in a home with great anxiety. I became conditioned to the addiction anxiety loop. That was my normal, I knew nothing else. It was what I tried, I learned and I searched for.

The roots of addiction and anxiety can show their face in such familiar places, usually right in our homes, our supposed safe zones. Remember, many addictions are learned behaviours as young children. We search to emulate those that care for us. We don't know what is right or wrong and can't choose from an early age. Combine that with certain genes and you have a miracle mix, needing only water and sunshine to grow. My family was no exception.

My mother was a perpetual bucket of nerves. She always thought the world was going to fall down around her. It doesn't help that she chose to spend her time reinforcing negative stimulus in her environment. Watching the news and focusing on negative events or gossip just aggravated her existence. Every small, little negative thing in her world was the END of the world. This is how she perceived it.

My mother just couldn't let go and get in the flow. She often aimed at managing her anxiety by eating, playing the piano, which she would practice for hours, or through educational achievement. My mother was a BRAINIAC! I love her so much and it's the reason why I am such a great doctor because she instilled in me the value of learning as much as you can and sharing it. She also instilled in me the maladaptive tool of both anxiety and fearing the worst as well as using food to calm down. It is there the addiction cycle began in my life.

Addictions are contagious, not only in the sense that those you raise will take on your habits, but also as one addiction is a gateway to another. The only time in my mother's life that I saw her manage her anxiety without those three outlets of food, piano or educational achievement, was a brief period of time that she became addicted to my Super Mario Brothers computer game. My sister and I would show up from school and there mother would be, on the living room floor beating my high score, and so enthralled in the game that you couldn't get her out of it.

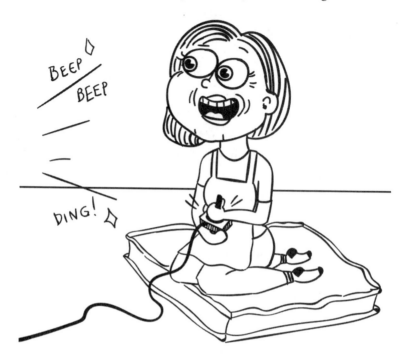

My mother's body responded to the anxiety and stress by being chronically constipated her entire life. I don't remember a time that she didn't comment on needing prunes or something to make her "correr", the Spanish verb for run, meaning run to the bathroom. In Traditional Chinese Medicine, the picture of constipation is correlated to being unable to let things go. This is very apparent in my mother. Her heightened anxiety and need to control extends beyond her mind and into her D-Spot. Yours does this too.

As my mother outwardly displays her anxiety, my father on the other hand, has an inner, more quiet anxiety. He learned to manage quite well by tending to his garden and working on his machinery which was a very well adaptive way to modify his environment, to tone down the stress. Where he would feel the crunch was in his bowels. He has the most beautiful blue eyes my mother had ever seen. These were her words and I agree that I was blessed to inherit those eyes. However, with blue peepers comes a tendency towards irritable bowel with diarrhea. Blue eyed people have a weakness in their D-Spot; they let go too much. It's a pattern that I have seen in practice. It goes along with not having adequate stomach acid levels and low zinc and vitamin B12, which coincidently, are needed to help with creating stomach acid and a healthy gut lining.

My amazing parents weren't at fault. Like them, not only do I have it ingrained genetically into my DNA, but I grew up in an environment that supported the addiction anxiety loop state of being. That was what my normal looked like. Your genes are the road map, but your environment is the car that takes the trip.

To this day, I need to mind my tendency to slip into a "normal" state of anxiety. I have to work at it and be very disciplined with my quiet practices.

So if anxiety is all you have ever known as your normal, you will seek to maintain that level of normalcy. That's just human nature because that is your comfortable spot. This just opens the door for addiction, whether your vice is sugar, alcohol, food, work or sex, or maybe all of them. Not only are you getting the ill effects of the substance but also the ill effects of the anxiety that is superimposed over the addiction.

I feel and see in my practice that there are more constantly anxious people than any other health condition and it's one of the reasons why our D-Spots are so damaged. Anxiety creates a major cascade of stress hormones via the adrenergic system[33], such as adrenaline in the short term and cortisol in the longterm. These are constantly pumping through our veins, especially for those with D-Spot drama like irritable bowel syndrome[34]. Oh, Sh*t! If you're genetically predisposed to anxiety and addiction, then you need to do everything in your power to change your environment so that you can regain normalcy and reclaim your D-Spot.

Instinct and Intuition Loop

As the addiction anxiety loop repeats its infinite pattern, we realize that there are many reasons why this rhythm is tough to break. Perhaps it's not about breaking the loop, but modifying it into an adaptive pattern that can elevate our existence. Remember, addiction and anxiety both hold within them gifts, should we choose to accept them.

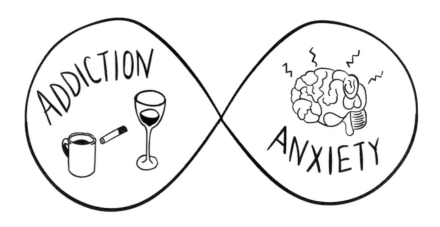

Addiction is so hard to break for many of us because in its primordial form, its essence is that of self care. It is an **instinct,** an instinct in some that is incredibly strong because of your genes. The GAD gene, which modulates the conversion of glutamate into gamma-aminobutyric acid (GABA), among others, is highly correlated to addiction[35] and anxiety[36]. When these genes malfunction, something known as a polymorphism, you produce little to no GABA, which is a neurotransmitter that makes you feel calm and well, and helps you to sleep. Unfortunately, you produce an excess of glutamate which is an excitatory neurotransmitter and has the opposite effect of GABA. You can imagine, that if you are low on GABA, you would look for substances like alcohol or marijuana that help you to create that feeling. There are other genes involved with the addiction anxiety infinity loop, but this is a predominant one that I see in myself, my family, and in many of my patients.

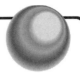

PEARL OF WISDOM

GENES CAN BE MODIFIED.

The environment will dictate whether genes are turned on or off. One must create the ideal environment if they wish to influence the expression of their genes. What's your environment?

This form of self care allows instant gratification to feel good. You don't feel good and you know that, so you search for the easiest and quickest fix. This is very normal. This is how we have evolved and survived through treacherous times, by listening to what we need. We look for the path of least resistance, the easiest way out.

Ask Yourself Right Now

Do you think you have addictions, either chemical, behavioural or with food? Do you have an addictive personality? Are you prone to anxiety? These are always such difficult questions to ask yourself. They take courage, but they are incredibly important answers to know.

Addiction is fed by feeling uncomfortable in your own skin and how you are living. That's why the addiction anxiety loop can become so strong and overpowering. Ask any addict. They all believe that they are in control of their addictions; they can stop whenever they want to. The reality is, they can't, and when they try, the process is arduous. It can literally rip their insides out. Trying to withhold their fix whether it's food, alcohol, cigarettes, sex or excess work, is excruciating. The more they restrict, the more anxious they get, and the more they want it. Self-medication is bound to occur the more anxious you get. Initially you feel good when you indulge, but as the effects wear off, you need more to keep you in a good, balanced state.

Your addictions are instinctual, whereas your anxiety is actually a call from your higher self, your **INTUITION**. Your anxiety elevates and increases the less you listen to your higher self, which only serves to perpetuate the cycle of addiction.

Instinct is raw! It is the evolutionary emotional command from the limbic system situated in the hypothalamic pathway in the middle of our brains[37]. The part of our brain that drives intuition seems to be different, depending on the research. Some say it's driven by the orbitofrontal cortex, within the inferior frontal gyrus and the middle temporal gyrus[38]. Other research suggests it is within the right superior temporal cortex and the bilateral inferior parietal cortex[39]. Interestingly, my feeling is that it goes deeper than that. Intuition is love at the highest level. It is our connection to the one, the cosmic, the universe, God. No matter which way you package it, we feel our intuition in all of our tissues that are connected to the nervous system, primarily the skin, the gut and in many areas of the brain.

Your intuition is your unconscious gateway to your higher self that will guide you through all in life. It shows you the best, brightest path[40], the yes and no; it moves you towards enlightenment. Your instincts move you towards immediate safety and prevention from harm such as "I'm starving, there must be a famine! I should eat everything in sight right now!" This differs from your intuition which says, "This is all I need right now; this will nourish my body and make me feel well". The instinct is not all bad, as it is there to serve and protect us. It has been known to save us, especially since we are living in a society of 24 hours, 7 days a week of stress. But this is exactly why we have to work on tuning in and listening to our bodies, as stress and anxiety can block the voice of our intuition. So while our instincts may tell us, "Survive right now at any cost", the cost more often than not can be a damaged D-Spot and many times extends further than that.

Tune in to your intuition over your instincts for it is trying to tell you something. Take this as an example. You see a hot man walk by. Your instincts say "You should bang him. He would make great, beautiful offspring!" However, your intuition, in the pit of your stomach says, "Hold on here, you have made a commitment to someone. There is no way that you will break that commitment. It is just not who you want to be." Obviously, this is a pretty significant moral test, but nonetheless, an issue dealing with listening solely to the primitive part of who we are, as opposed to the spiritual part that is working onwards towards enlightenment. Now what if we correlated it to your food choices?

Your primordial instincts want sugar, sugar and more sugar with a little extra salt and fat to go with it. In fact, as I've mentioned before, you have been programmed (instinctually) to want, crave and seek out glorious sugar, salt and fat. It is our addictive instinct that has helped us to survive as a species[41]. Now your higher self, your intuition, knows that when there is a piece of pie vs. a plate of broccoli and chicken, one will better serve you.

It is not the instant gratification of a sugary piece of pie, but rather the nourishing, healthful plate of broccoli and chicken. Both will help you grow, one on your waistline, the other in a spiritual, emotional and nutritional way.

Your instinct is what connects you to animal species. See that, want that, get that. Your intuition is your higher self, the self that knows what is right, what is good, what is healthy. Take time and learn to distinguish between the want and the what is best for you. A practice of instinct vs. intuition and learning to discern the difference between the two will be a major step in making your D-Spot divine.

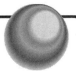

PEARL OF WISDOM

INSTINCT CAN BE CALMED. INTUITION CAN
BE CURATED.

The problem that you may be finding now is that you are very out of tune with your body and its signals. We are not observing natural laws, and most of us know it. Like me, I was feeling guilty about my addictions, not being coherent and showing myself one way to the world but acting a totally different way. Some of us choose to be completely oblivious to it. Something is out of whack in your life and you may not be able to pinpoint it. You just know something is not quite right. Perhaps you are not ready to listen to it.

Timing and Your D-Spot, Getting in Tune

How are we so out of tune? Our timing and natural cues are completely out of synchronicity with nature. So many people are disconnected to how they are feeling. Most can't even sense the divine sensation of being hungry. Some need to be taught how to sense their internal hunger by external cues[42]. We will learn this here.

When I ask patients, "Are you hungry?" most say, "I don't even know what hungry is. I eat because I'm supposed to." Many of us have listened and been brainwashed by the 'experts', who think they know more than we know about our own bodies. My response to this is, "Who in the bleep are 'they', these so-called experts?" You follow their plans and because of this, you end up suffering. You try to stay on these so-called health plans only to fail miserably. You tell yourself, "I have no willpower. I suck. Why can't I do anything right?" This negative self talk and perfectionist attitude just feeds your self hatred, more fuel for the fire. This puts you further into the ruts of despair. This further messes up your D-Spot. Being out of tune sets us up for breakdown in our metabolic system and sets the stage for diabetes and cancer[43]. If we are to improve our health, we must learn to listen to our bodies and tune in to our natural synchronicities and internal clocks.

No single expert has all of the answers, including myself. I'm a firm believer that you must try things out and pick the pieces that fit your puzzle. Keep on learning, never stop trying. Sometimes you pick up a gem and it all works for you. This book may very well be that gem for you; I may be your perfect guide. If that is so, go all in. Listen to your body. You will learn to trust it. In fact, it is difficult to go against every single cell of your body that contains mitochondria and genes that are clued in to environmental signals. The signals are all around for us to observe. You just need to be aware of what you are presently doing that may be perpetuating your disharmony and keeping you out of tune. Tuning in can elevate your life! **Intuition is key!**

Did you know that you do certain things at different times of the day because they are just instinctual at that time of the day? Many of our instinctual habits are stimulated by external cues. Many people don't realize that all the cells of our bodies are governed by the same natural laws[44]. These natural laws dictate how we sleep, what we want and crave to eat, and what time of the day or month we like to get frisky.

These patterns and rhythms of nature are regulated by three types of clocks known as circadian (24 hrs periods), ultradian (less than 24 hrs) and infradian (more than 24 hrs) which are all directed by nature and certain stimulus.

Life is all about timing, and timing has triggers and cues such as a wink of the eye here, a toss of the hair there. Get it? Got it. Let's move on.

The cues that come from the outside such as your exposure to light, electrical magnetic frequencies, what you see and feel, what you eat and drink, and the bugs that get into your body are all external conductors that are known as zeitgebers. Fun name!

Zeitgebers conduct much of our biology. These exogenous cues synchronize our internal clocks and processes. These cues stimulate our internal messengers, like neurotransmitters, hormones and immune modulators, hence, exerting a biological effect on the body. As an example, our skin changes according to the cues delivered by our environment[45].

Light is one of the best known zeitgebers. It is our external clock. Light tells us when to wake and when to sleep. It signals the receptors in our skin and eyes and tells the pineal gland to produce melatonin, to get a great night of sleep.

The problem is that often we are exposed to an overabundance of artificial light at all times of the day, including right before we go to bed. You may harmlessly be looking at your iPhone or Android and not realize that this is majorly affecting your sleep processes and production of melatonin[46], messing up your circadian rhythm and increasing your risk for mood alternations[47] and diseases such as cancer[48]. Breast cancer patients are known to have higher rates of circadian rhythm dysfunction than the normal population[49].

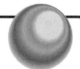

PEARL OF WISDOM

A common prescription in my practice is to purchase blue-blocking glasses, especially for those kids who are having problems sleeping at night or who play a plethora of video games. The orange glasses block out the blue light from electronic screens, therefore reducing any interference with melatonin production before bed.

Electromagnetic pollution such as wifi, electrical, cell phone towers and signals can also disrupt our day night rhythms balance[50]. This zeitgeber acts via an electrical sine wave which is a signal that disrupts natural cellular function. Each cell has an automatic death switch. When replication goes severely wrong, cells lose their ability to know when to hit the terminate button, which is the precursor to dysplastic cells[51].

How do these things affect our D-Spot? It's no shocker that your appetite, without a good night's rest, increases, and you have a tendency to eat more calories[52]. Does this mean that shutting off the lights and putting away the phones, gadgets and computers could make you have a happier D-Spot and possibly lose weight? It sure does, so why not? Reducing your screen time will help you regulate your whole system.

A very interesting example of another external cue is that of **facial mimicry**[53]. This was at one time an evolutionary advantage. Our neurological system sees and mimics facial expressions, making us feel like who we are looking at. If one of your caveman friends would have a look of fear on his face, this would create fear in you and signal you to run away from the threat. Now, this scenario is no longer the norm and it just perpetuates a tragic state of living a life in fear, unless you're one of those who chooses to always wear a smile.

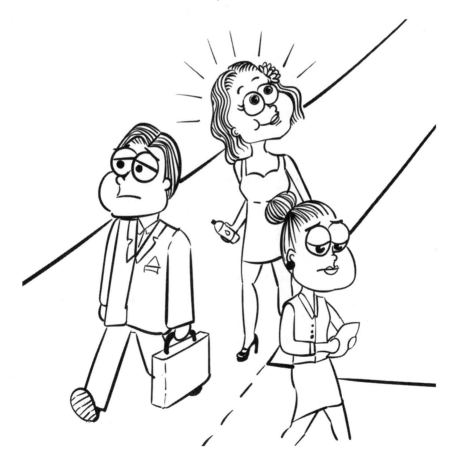

Since facial expressions are contagious, it comes as no surprise that mood would be contagious as well, known in academic circles as **emotional contagion**. Nowadays, this zeitgeber serves us to perpetuate the problems of our modern day society, unless you have chosen to surround yourself with only positive people. The pain cues from the external faces of friends, family and colleagues create a society that is relishing in depression, anxiety and loss of passion.

We must be vigilant of the cues that we expose ourselves to, as they conduct our internal orchestra. We must choose with what and whom we want to surround ourselves. Will you have the lights and wifi on all night? Will you hang around someone whose emotions make you miserable? Or do you choose to change your practices and cleanse the toxic Debbie Downers for a better life of passionate, happy people?

As you know, our **thoughts** control our actions and intentions. Thoughts are often stimulated by external zeitgebers, something you saw or something that someone told you. We are so interconnected and interdependent with our environment, it's no wonder that when people are locked up in an isolation room, they go crazy. They lose all of their external cues, what entrains them. We need to be guided ideally to feel great and elated, and hopefully to not feel flat like a tire.

Food is another important external cue and hence like light, one of the most important biological messengers that dictates how our bodies act. Did you know that your entire internal gut environment begins to change within 24hrs of adopting healthier practices[54]? Hyper caloric and highly palatable foods can be such a strong zeitgeber, that short term wanting can easily become an entrenched addiction[55]. If you eat a diet high in saturated fats, processed full of sugar and salt, you are not only changing the environment in your gut but also in your brain, and sadly not for your benefit. With a changing environment in your gut, the bacteria that comes from the outside changes. A healthy gut environment means healthy gut bacteria. An unhealthy gut means unhealthy bugs.

Since our guts are an external environment on our insides, the population of gut bacteria that is living in our intestines are also classified as zeitgebers. Depending on what we feed our bodies and gut bacteria, these little critters feast as much as we do. We change our internal environment because these critters will produce either noxious chemicals, or good things like vitamins, that make us feel great.

In addition, some yeasts actually make us crave more sugar by sending out signals. Think back to a time you may have had to take antibiotics. I know that for me, each time I have taken them, I am diligent about taking probiotics in between doses. Still, I get a savage craving for sugar that is difficult to satisfy. Often times I become plagued with maybe a yeast infection or two. It takes time, good quality food and great probiotics to make my internal signalling shift, to change the environment on my insides that are created from the outside!

Supplements are also a form of external zeitgebers that cue and entrain the system to do certain things. From the outside, we can change our insides, and we see the results as the change comes from the inside to manifest on the outside.

It's incredible to see that there are so many external factors that affect how in tune we are with our insides. If you think it's only the good things that entrain our bodies, think again. Drugs of abuse also entrain the rhythms of our body[56]. The external affects our internal environments and the hormones, neurotransmitters and immune modulators that flood our system. Remember that our bodies are a complex system of ebb and flow. For every action, there is an equal and opposite reaction. This is one of Newton's laws, but is also mimicked by the traditional asian philosophy of yin and yang. For every light there is darkness, for every happiness there is sadness. Everything is equally and oppositely created.

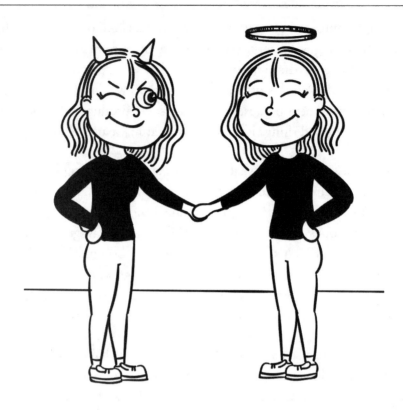

When the Rhythms are in Tune, Your Orchestra can Play

All of this is not new knowledge. It is just simply not being utilized to its full extent, not being adopted for our better being. Don't you think it's time to embody it now? To get in flow with your outside environment and perhaps tweak it to be more natural, especially in your daily life. Getting in tune takes time and practice. But getting in tune will help you to discover more of what you really want and less of what you are gravitating towards because your body feels that it needs it. After all, isn't that the basis of an addiction and feeling uncomfortable in your skin?

Accept

Feeling good in your own skin isn't always easy to do. With anxiety and addiction and not being able to tune in to our environments, we can feel more like an alien in our bodies. We have to work at reframing how we think about what is afflicting us. For me, the gift of my anxiety is that it makes me a person who is incredibly intuitive, being able to tune into the zeitgebers of my world, as long as I'm present and working towards that goal. If I'm mindless and numbing my feelings, I won't know left from right. This intuition is incredible when I'm mindful and quiet. It just flows through me, fuels my creativity and all sorts of wonderful thoughts.

Being intuitive isn't all butterflies and roses for there are thorns too. When you are intuitive, you feel others' pain and you tap into not only the good things, but you feel it all. Sometimes those feelings can just be so overwhelming. Remember that it's not just your stuff you zone into, it's also everything and everyone around you too. It can be a lot. Some of us choose to numb it and walk away, instead of simply accept it. Get good with the gifts, just like you need to get good with the daily grind, which we will talk about shortly.

Choose

Part of taking on any new health practice is to learn to work and get better at listening to your gut, A.K.A. D-Spot, and to take a moment to make a choice. Do not repeat the patterns that you so easily fall into. Addiction keeps you in a non-empowered state, a state of fear, a state of not being able to live without the substance. Freedom from addiction gives you exactly that, pure utter freedom, a freedom to live well, to not need anything more than is necessary, just you and all that has created you.

Freedom requires two things, awareness and discipline. Only with true awareness of the moment and your inner workings, can you choose what and who you want to be, and how you want to feel. Yes, you can choose how you feel, from your D-Spot to your mind. Making the choice to explore how you are presently feeling in your innards will enlighten your every moment. Choice is the divine gift. Choice is what separates us from other mammals. We do not run solely on our primitive brains and our instincts, "Grrr, I want this and not that".

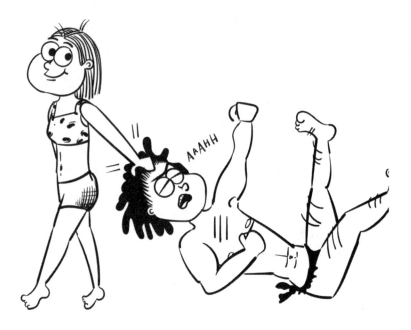

Your prefrontal cortex, your instinct, can decide if this or that is what we want for our life. Let it be your guide.

You always have a choice. Choose to listen to both your inspired instinct and to your divine intuition, and work towards evolving towards your higher self consistently. That is the way to a divine D-Spot. Take my hand let's go there together.

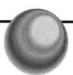

PEARL OF WISDOM

DIFFERENTIATING INSTINCT & INTUITION

Instict: Quick onset, propels you to act now – impulsively.
Intuition: It takes time to manifest and develop. Trusting your D-Spot over time will improve your ability to have faith in your intuition. Trust yourself. You know the right choice & the journey you should choose.

CHAPTER 3

THE DIVINE IN OUR DIGESTION

"Your mind is your master, so mind your
master and then master your mind."

-Dr. Marisol

Digestion is divine, our D-Spot is our link to the divine, to our being in flow. Why? It's where we digest life. It's how we nourish ourselves, both from a nutrient micromolecular and macromolecular perspective, down to the way we take on emotional trials and tribulation.

In this chapter we are going to explore the functionality and physiology of the D-Spot. But before getting into the nitty gritty of how the D-Spot works, it's important to note that even though the D-Spot is mechanical in its operation, its job is to take large pieces and break, grind and macerate them down to smaller digestible pieces.

If you look at any philosopher of life, high performance coach, positive psychologist or guru, they all recommend to take things in smaller pieces and break them down so that they are "easier to digest". This is one of the reasons why digestive health is so fundamental to our well being. If we are unable to get 'good' with how we grind the basic molecules of life and if we live within the realm of addiction and anxiety, then we are unable to listen to our intuition and instinct. Why? It's because our guts are so muddled with food and we are literally putting garbage into our gutters. How can we live in peace?

Before stepping into the physiology and learning how the gut interconnects with all of our systems, there are four priming concepts we need to cover.

1. The Gift Within The Grind

2. Discipline Indulgence Principle

3. The D-Spot, Your Agent Of Change

4. Novelty Now

These concepts will set the stage for your mindset moving forward. So to say, we will baste your brain to prepare you for the steps to come. After all, your mind is your master, so mind your master and you will master your mind.

The Gift Within The Grind

When our D-Spot is not divine, it is in quite a grind.

As you've learnt, our addictions take up space in our minds. They take up valuable, precious real estate that we don't want to lose. The science of neuroplasticity points to entrenched neuropathways related to reward in addiction[57]. The more that you repeat the behaviours, the deeper entrenched they become, in regards to binging or overindulging in a certain type of food that may not be good for you. These entrenched pathways make it difficult to change, but not impossible. There is no running away from an addiction. The only way is to accept that choosing change may feel much like grinding down a rock initially, but through the process, you will reveal precious gems. It's arduous, but totally worth it.

The ironic thing is that the addict is searching for escape, because the addiction becomes a grind as well. No matter what the addiction, it allows escape. Within the binge, the addict finds a fake freedom, a moment of numbness, a moment where all is well and there is no pain, no pressure, just pleasure. Once the cycle is done, the addict searches for the numbing and it is within this space the addict is caged by his/her addiction. The only way out is to stop numbing oneself. You must become present to the here and the now. You must feel the pain and go through the stages of healing the emotional pain, no different than physical pain.

I find it so incredibly amazing that many patients are at the end of their ropes, so sick of being sick and tired. Before I start delivering my advice, I ask them, "Are you willing to do anything and everything to get better, to get out of the vicious cycle that you are in?"

I know that it takes practice, and practice can become work, which enhances the feeling that your daily grind is way more grinding than it should be. However, I need to mentally prepare them for that.

Patients often state, "I will do anything you ask me doc, anything."

They always answer with such resolve, so set that they can, and will, do anything.

In return I advise, "Great, I want you to switch your morning coffee to green tea."

Nine out of ten patients will look at me in awe and object.

They reply, "Oh no, not that. I can't live without my coffee, it's not that I'm addicted to the coffee doc, it's just that I love the taste."

To which I say, "Well you told me that you would do anything it takes, and if it takes switching from coffee to tea, why won't you do that? If you want to get better, you will do whatever it takes, won't you? At least that's what you said, and giving up coffee isn't exactly giving up your first born child... or is it? It isn't like giving up oxygen or water.

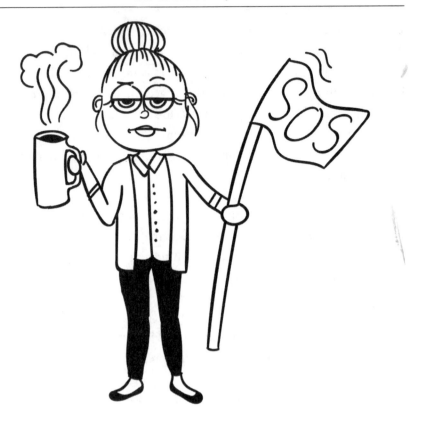

Coffee you can live without, even if you like the taste. Hey, I like cigarettes, but I know I can live without them."

This may sound a bit harsh, but I want my patients to think. I've lived in the downhill grind of being controlled by substances, thinking I can't be apart from them and I chose differently. I want to instill that in my patients.

So, if one can entrench neurological pathways for behaviours that are addictive, is it then possible to un-trench them and create new **freedom pathways**? Yes, you can create new neuronal networks with practice, lots of practice. Practice is the mother of all skills.

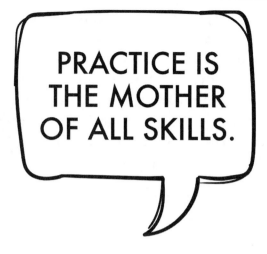

PRACTICE IS
THE MOTHER
OF ALL SKILLS.

You are so good at your maladaptive behaviours because you practise them daily.

You practise your addictions daily, so why can't you practise like a baby, an Olympian, a master musician? Why can't you retrain yourself to have different behaviours? You absolutely can, it's called positive plastic change, and novelty will be your friend in this process[58]. Like a baby taking its first steps, novelty increases your epinephrine which helps with entrenching new neuronal networks. It just takes baby steps, and you have to be okay with the process of change. I like to call it the gift within the grind. It's good hard work. It takes constant focus, but that's what it takes, and that's what you are going to deliver. Period. You are going to promise yourself that.

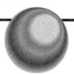

PEARL OF WISDOM

To create a new neuronal network you need a little epinephrine, a little excitement, & a little dopamine. So sit up, change up, do a little something that spikes your cortisol. Get up from where you are sitting. These things will pump your blood pressure and with that, your epinephrine. Voila, a new neuronal network is made.

Think of it like this, a gem stone isn't a gemstone until the rough hard surfaces of rock that encapsulate it are ground and filed away to display a gorgeous semi-precious stone. Then, detailed grinding and shaving work follows to make it a gem. Life is no different. We must grind down the rough, and it might be painful, to reveal the true treasure. When you are in the grind of addiction, you don't get a gem at the end of the grind. But when it's a health practice, you get diamonds. Get good with the daily grind. It's worth it, you're worth it!

I love castor oil packs so much and one of the reasons is because they promote dopamine production, helping to create new health practices and break bad habits. We will talk more on this later.

If you see yourself as very habitual, with addictions that you think you will never let go of, stop, and get a reality check. You CAN, you can do anything you want to! You just need to want it badly enough and then you have to do the work to get it. You need to be conscious of your actions; you need to be here, right here, right now, nowhere else. You need to absorb what is being laid before you. Take note of the plan and start right now. Don't wait. **It takes guts to go deep.**

Discipline Indulgence Principle

If freedom is to be achieved, you cannot be chained to a set of rules. My principle of practice is that of discipline and indulgence. Strict discipline is required when the going gets tough and you aren't feeling well. This is not the time to be indulgent, but the time to abide by natural laws so that you can heal. Remember, time to tune in!

There is, however, a time for indulgence, and without it we wouldn't have a balanced life. Balancing your life and creating true freedom is about working within the Discipline Indulgence Principle. Discipline helps to create true indulgences. Ironic, but true.

Take this as an example. In most cases, if you have a sensitivity to a food, your body will react with inflammation, irritation and overall stress in your gut and body when you consume the food. You simply cannot continue to consume the food forever, as it will continue to irritate and affect you more. Every individual has a different time of tolerance, meaning they can tolerate it for a period of time without consequence, but suddenly it affects them. All individuals who are sensitive to a certain food need to give their beautiful body a break so that it can rest and recuperate. It's no different from when you have the flu. You must rest and recuperate in order to feel better.

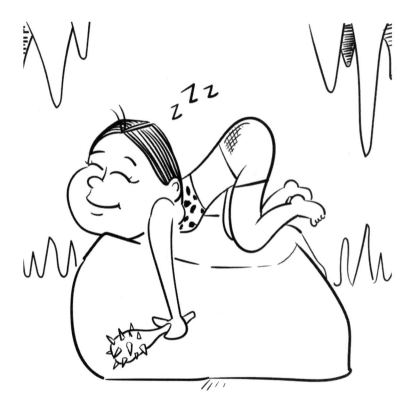

When ready, in most cases you can indulge in it again. You will feel it but at least you are aware. Some people such as those with Celiac disease, which is an allergy to gluten, simply can never introduce the food. Others can introduce and "indulge" in the food from time to time and it won't cause the physical stress that it once did. Ah, the taste of freedom, literally.

Indulgences from time to time make our discipline livable and real. When you are disciplined, you open up the space to allow indulgence. During this book experience there will be periods of discipline that will open up your world of indulgence. Find your balance, so that your life is full of all types of experiences.

The D-Spot, the Agent of Change

Why are we so afraid of change? Why do we like things to be as they are? Simply put, it is because we are all creatures of habit. The only problem is right now your habits are creating an unhealthy D-Spot, and this is a huge dilemma. We must start to change one by one, habits and practices that are contributing to the dilemma of the D-Spot. The funny thing is, our survival depends on being flexible, on being open to change and our D-Spot is one of our biggest agents of change in our body. It is the master of experiencing newness and change.

Because the D-Spot is that divine place where the outside meets your insides, the change required for improvement is multi-faceted. The D-Spot is the connection of all that is us. **It connects our moods and mind[59], our immune system and gut[60], our hormones and health[61] and our nourishment from both a physical and psychological level. It's how we intake the world and also how we let go.**

It is the hub of our bodies. It is the main attraction and why we must all learn to be in harmony with our D-Spots.

The D-Spot is so important to our health, that when we have it in divine shape, we are WELL. When it is out of balance we are all wrong. The first part of healing any condition is to ensure that your D-Spot is functioning and healthy. If you treat your body without caring for your D-Spot, you will never get better.

Everything begins from within.

Change will come from your focus on you. The incredible part is that when you work at changing your D-Spot, something miraculous happens. The change from within reflects in your expression. What you feel inside, you will manifest on the outside. The beauty building within vibrates all around you and can be felt by others.

The best example of this is when a patient presents at my clinic with skin conditions. I know that their D-Spot is damaged and deranged due to the lifestyle they are living[62] but they have no clue. They apply topical lotions and potions in mass amounts, all to no avail. The skin is one of the messengers of the D-Spot.

Those with depression express sadness and lack of lustre on their faces. Their depressive moods drag them down and deny them joy. The mind is my messenger. You can see the health of your gut on your skin and in how your mind works[63]. When you feel better in your D-Spot, you are better and you live better. You simply glow from a physical perspective and vibe from a mental perspective.

We need to look at change as something good, and come to the realization that change is the only thing that will ever remain the same. It's natural in every way and is expressed over and over again in the patterns in our lives. As we are born, we go through stages of change from birth to babe, from infant to child, from teenager to adult, from adult to elder, and ultimately dying and turning into dust. Such are the stages of life and the natural evolution of change.

The unbelievable thing is that we are programmed for change. Did you know that in seven years, every single cell of your body will turn over? You won't be the same you, as you were seven years ago. We evolve, and our evolution is one step at a time, one hour, one day, one year, one decade, one century, one civilization, one era.

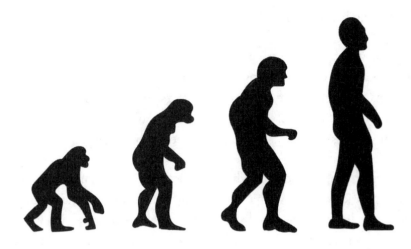

Change comes and we have no other option but to accept it. Our DNA says so[64], as does Brendon Burchard, motivational and high performance coach extraordinaire explains, "Either you choose to change yourself or something else will force you to change. Either become the agent of change or allow yourself to be a victim of change."

You decide that you want to feel better, you want to feel vibrant, you want to live every moment to its fullest. This is your train of thought. This needs to be your mantra, "Enough is enough, I want to live my life. I am here and I am vibrant. Life is too short to wait for something to change me. I can change, I can do this".

And if you think you are too old to change, think again. We are never too old for anything. There are countless examples of people who have changed the world at an old age such as Mother Theresa, Gandhi and Nelson Mandela.

Imagine these people and their ability to be flexible like water, to be ever-changing and evolving for the better. They are creators of major change in both their inside and outside worlds! Everything is interconnected, and when you ignite a change internally, you can really reignite your life externally and bring your true gifts to this world.

The other option is that you wait for something to change you. Usually that something is huge, such as a cancer diagnosis, where you finally quit smoking, albeit sometimes too late. Your life partner dies tragically and you decide to never again be such an angry person in a relationship and to treat your partner better. These are all examples of it being too late. There is an excellent saying that embodies this problem, "People don't change when they see the light, they change when they get burnt." (Unknown author)

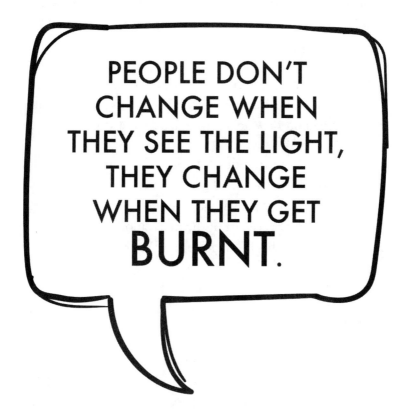

Don't fall victim to this thought pattern because you do not need to live by it. You can change when you see the light, you just have to choose it. Choose to live in the light and not within the fire.

Usually if you wait for something from the outside to change you, it's typically something of astronomical proportions that has major detrimental effects on your life. I've seen this most often when someone comes to a naturopathic doctor's office after being diagnosed with cancer. Or worse, they come after multiple rounds of treatment that have all failed. Then, and only then, do they decide that they are willing to work to change their lifestyle and practices that are both contributing to their disease, or also contributing to the drugs not working.

When talking about the D-Spot, it's the area of your body that is programmed for the fastest change. No, you don't need to wait seven years to have a new D-Spot. In fact, changes are noted as quickly as 24 hours after changing your diet.

The D-Spot is the body's agent of change. Its function is to change things that are coming into our lives and our job is to be like the D-Spot, to be in good flow, to allow and accept change.

What is the best way to introduce change into your life? To start, do something a little different everyday. Get in the practice and habit of doing things differently. This will help you to regain flexibility and to feel renewed energy. This is part of the motivation[65]. Be like water, get in flow. Get into it and begin to grow, now. Your D-Spot does it every day. Get in flow with your D-Spot.

Novelty Now

Habits and practice can either lead to our demise or to an amazing destiny. To not let our habits ruin our fruitful lives, we must consistently be implementing change and novelty. Novelty practices are the first step to breaking fixed maladaptive patterns. They also make you more accustomed to change and allows you to be more flexible, more resilient to stressors. But this being said, only if you practise them!

When you are rigid, like rock or stone, you may seem so strong, so put together. The reality is that you are more likely to get worn down and eventually be broken. When rigid and strong, soft things become major stressors and this regular occurrence puts more and more weight, so to say, on your shoulders. At one point, you will break. Natural laws say so, so does Chinese philosopher Lao Tzu. In the Tao he recommends for you to be like water, to flow.

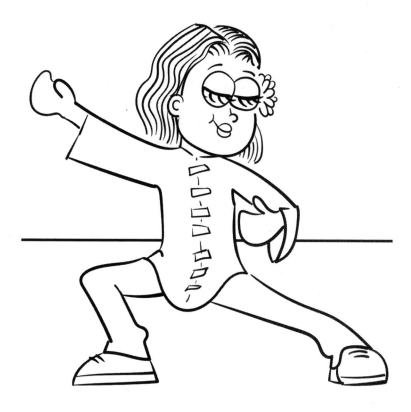

Water works with resistance and does not work against it. Over control of ones life leads to unnecessary stress. When you control, you repeat the same patterns because they are known, and when things don't go as planned, stress is often experienced. Stress is the ultimate villain, who was once a friend.

The next time you go to get gas, go to a new gas station. Dine out at a different restaurant. Go on holiday in a different place. Don't do an all-inclusive but actually book and plan a trip. Newness adds excitement. It adds a different kind of stress, known as eu-stress, a term created by Dr. Hans Seyle, a McGill researcher and father of the stress theory. It's still stress, so sometimes too much 'new' all at once can negatively impact you. But when you add little doses of eu-stress into your life practice, it leads to incredible results, including feelings of wellbeing and the spirit of excitement and challenge. Plus, you develop those new neuronal networks in your brain that we spoke about.

The same principle applies when new patients come to see me (with the exception of those with a deadly disease where everything needs to be radically changed right away because time is of the essence). I have patients implement a few new novelty health practices all beginning with the D-Spot, and I build upon them. Go to the appendix to see my top five tools for your health practice (all included in the Queen Kit). To be successful, patients need to understand the interconnectedness of their D-Spot and their health. This is much like the experience of this book and our online programs. You can ultimately save thousands of dollars at the naturopathic doctor's office. Many of these things you can do on your own and your doctor will serve to guide you deeper, where it can be difficult to go alone. Go check out our kit, our online preferred programs and sign up for our weekly show at www.drmarisol.com.

Now how is our D-Spot so interconnected?

Food and Mood

Food creates your mood and that's why the potential for addiction to food is so high. Mood-based disorders are one of the biggest problems plaguing our society today. Interestingly enough, the rise in mood-based disorders coincides with the increased processing and addition of sugar to our food, the increasing genetic modification of our food, and microwave use. It seems, in terms of food, we are going backwards. The quality of our food is decreasing, yet the quantity is increasing. Why is that? Simply, because low quality malnourishing food does not fill us up. In fact, you can eat a lower calorie, high-nutrient diet and feel less hungry[66]. High caloric, nutrient-void food does not give us what we need to fuel our D-Spot. It is dead food, so to say. So we crave and crave and crave because our body, mind and soul are missing something. What they are missing is true nourishment. Food is an element that creates your mood, and it can affect it in more ways than one.

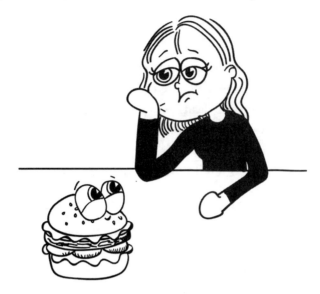

If you feed yourself low vitality food, food that is low in nutrients and low in enzymes, or perhaps has been nuked to literally radiate out whatever nutrition was left in the food, you end up feeling low energy. Low vitality food equals a low vitality person - a pretty simple concept. If you are lacking the macro and micromolecules to make your body and brain work well, how can you feel good? It's no different than when someone is anemic or low in iron. They will feel fatigued and lethargic. So too will you, if you are lacking these substances.

The other aspect is that in certain foodstuffs, certain molecules mimic our own bodies' chemical messengers and can wreak havoc on our bodies' balance mechanisms. Take dairy and wheat as examples. As discussed before, certain proteins in these substances actually create an opiate analogue.

Yes that's right, opiates - substances that are highly addictive and make you feel good while you take them, but once they wear off, you crash. It's likely one of the many reasons why we are so addicted to dairy and wheat, not to mention we have made such a habit of eating these foods.

Food, from an evolutionary perspective, is meant to make us feel good. Feeling good is what tells us that we are satisfied, that we have had enough. This is an incredibly important part of food and nutrition. It is meant to make us feel good. However, these days, we seem to feel less than satisfied with both our lives and our food.

Another aspect of mood being regulated by food is the supreme sugar and caffeine highs and lows. We use these substances to keep us going, often when we have tight deadlines. I too, commonly hear, "I need coffee to get going in the mornings." Nothing irks me more than seeing someone have a Coke for breakfast. It's the all-magical, two-in-one, sugar with a spot of caffeine. Sounds much like it's a close friend of coffee.

Our D-Spot is so tightly connected to our mood, that as I have said before, many of its processes are regulated by neurotransmitters similar to those that are in the brain, like nitric oxide, serotonin and dopamine. You can't separate your mood from your D-Spot health for they are one and the same. In fact, a great doctor will first rule out D-Spot problems with patients if they have depression or anxiety. There could be a multitude of issues from deficiencies due to poor absorption, food sensitivities, dysbiosis in the gut, and more. You will learn all about the major culprits of the D-Spot and how they affect the body in the next chapter.

D-Spot Drama - Who's Hormonal Now?

Since our D-Spot is the outside on our inside, it can be a very moody system. It can definitely have its own form of PMS. Its job is to feel the outside, on our insides, and if this is disrupted, it gets completely deranged, and I mean MAD deranged. Shall I dare say, it can become 'hormonal'.

Our D-Spots are truly sensitive creatures. The D-Spot is our second brain and it literally has a mind of its own. It's just like the saying, "Most men think with their second head." In this case, our second head is in our D-Spot. When you feel butterflies in your stomach, you are essentially feeling the stress and anxiety of a situation.

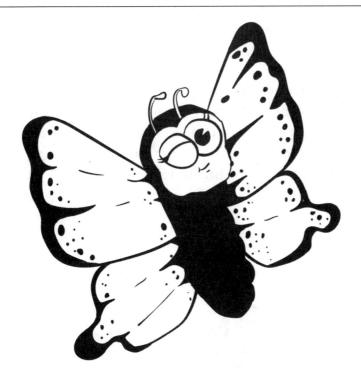

Perhaps the unease that you are feeling is not from your mind, but from your gut. As a society and culture, we have painted it as little butterflies, batting their wings in our belly. It's that frantic sensation that we don't know how to handle. It's just one of the signs that our guts begin to deliver. Listening in to the sensations that we get from our gut delivers an enormous amount of messages to us.

As an example, female and male patients with irritable bowel syndrome (IBS) experience it very differently. Why? It's because in females, ovarian hormones modulate gastrointestinal functions. It's not the causing factor of the IBS, it's just one of the ways that transit time of the D-Spot is affected[67]. Our guts are hormonal. This is also why more women are plagued with D-Spot drama than men.

The D-Spot is truly divine, standing alone on its own merits, yet completely intertwined with all of the most important regulatory systems of the body, including the immune system.

D-Spot and Immunity

The immune system is the guardian of our temple and our D-Spot. It is the armed forces of our body and is found all over, but most concentrated on our outsides, both near our skin and of course in our D-Spot, the outside that is in our inside. I like to think of the immune system as our great defender. It's the superhero of the body, fighting for what is right and what is just, helping to keep the peace and calmness in our systems.

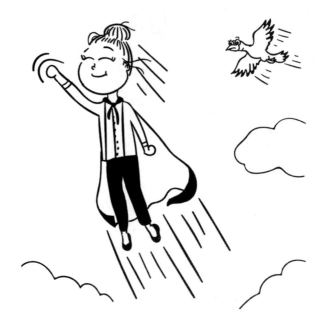

The immune system is in its greatest concentration at the D-Spot. Why is this? This is because it's the spot in our body where we intake the most from the outside world and with that, there is the greatest risk of invasion. So, the defenses must be set up there.

The immune system is divided into both first line (innate), and second line (adaptive) of defense. The first line is mainly mechanical, such as barriers like the skin or stomach acid that are non-specific, meaning they block it all out. The second line is based on an intricate system of defense, where identity matters. Our immune system identifies the invader and creates super soldiers specialized to attack that invader.

We need to avoid treating our D-Spots like a big old dump truck, placing all types of bad food in there to stress it out.

When we are stressed, we deplete our immune system[68]. True also, when we over do it with sugar[69]. One teaspoon of sugar will decrease your immune system activity for five hours. Consider that 250mL of apple juice contains ten teaspoons of sugar or 250mL of orange juice contains six teaspoons of sugar. Imagine the amount of sugar that we consume daily. We are constantly not allowing our immune system to do its job. Unfortunately, we overwhelm our army and a consequence of this can be that our superheroes stop fighting the bad guys, or worse, can become mutinous and rebel against our own body. That's what an autoimmune condition is; your body begins attacking itself.

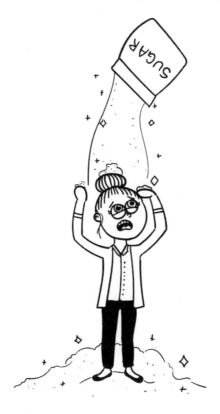

Eau de Throne™ is a tool included in the Queen Kit that I love to use with patients to support their immune response (as well as the castor oil pack!). It is a medicinal, all-natural and organic After You Poo Parfum™ bathroom deodorizer spray that contains organic essential oils which help to calm the nervous system, balance hormones, kill bad bacteria in the air and improve the immune system.

The Job of a Healthy D-Spot

The majority of us are living with a destroyed D-Spot that simply doesn't have the ability to do its job properly. Its job is to break down, digest, assimilate, absorb and eliminate.

When damage occurs in the D-Spot, which will be the subject of the next chapter, it reacts in a few ways. Many of you have probably heard of the book Gut, by Giulia Enders, which is a good generalization for the multitude of things that are occurring in an unhealthy gut. There is also an immune battle. There is inflammation, there is loss of a healthy gut lining and there is loss of a healthy mucous protective barrier. Also, there is a disrupted environment in terms of bad bugs versus good bugs, and yes, there is leaking of the intestinal membrane. Sh*t has just hit the fan!

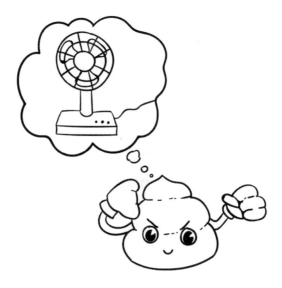

The D-Spot is the big game changer and it creates BIG change. It takes a substance, manipulates it, and changes it into something digestible and absorbable. Then it takes what's left, along with the bad byproducts of said substance, and eliminates it out of the body. This is vital to our life. Change is the only thing that remains constant in life. As such, your D-Spot is the master of change and needs to remain in constant flow. It needs flow in order to go. What comes in, must go out, and ideally it flows in and out with ease.

The Big Three - Mechanical Jobs of the D-Spot

1. Digestion

Digestion is one of the most important parts of life. We must digest life in all of its aspects. From food to relationships to emotions, it's all part of digestion. It's why the D-Spot is so interconnected with your intuition and your emotions.

Digestion takes outside stimulus (i.e. food stuff) and mechanically and chemically breaks it down into molecules that we can absorb into our bodies. It all begins, not in our stomachs, but actually in our nose, eyes[70], mouths and our minds. You think about a delicious piece of cheesy pizza and you start to salivate.

I always like to look to Mother Nature for examples of these natural instincts in action. I look at my little Yorkie, Lola. The minute she sees and smells food, usually my dinner or something I am making, she starts to lick her lips. She can't help it. She is salivating. That is step one of the digestive process. The senses becoming tantalized by food.

The next step is the mechanical breakdown as food reaches our mouths. Ideally, you have pre-mechanically broken it down with your fork and your knife, or broken that piece of bread with your hands. Your teeth do a smashing job with the food, mechanically breaking it down to mush, that is only if you chew on it for long enough. Many of us forget this vital part of digestive hygiene and inhale our food, which gives our D-Spots more and more work to do.

Use our Queen of the Thrones™ Grateful Dung™ bracelet included in the Queen Kit to help with thorough chewing, using each Tiger's eye bead to represent one chew. The bracelet also doubles as a tool for implementing a simple gratitude practice before meals, to relax your gut and ease it into the 'rest and digest' parasympathetic state. More on this later.

Now the other aspect of mechanical breakdown is saliva. Saliva contains both enzymes and bacteria. The enzymes are salivary amylase, produced in the salivary glands that commence the breakdown of carbohydrates and sugars in the mouth, and lingual lipase, that begins the breakdown of fats. The bacteria also serve to begin breakdown of food, but to a lesser extent. One of the keys to good digestion is that the environment of the mouth is alkaline. In an alkaline environment, both fats and carbohydrates can break down. So the face time, so to say, that the food gets in the mouth, exposes it not only to mechanical breakdown but also to chemical breakdown via the enzymes and bacteria. Throughout the D-Spot, in fact, you will be seeing and learning about the various combinations of mechanical and chemical breakdown.

Once that piece of delicious pizza gets swallowed down the black hole that is the esophagus, it should look quite differently than what it did when it was a piece of pie. It should be a form of mush that slips and slides down the lubricated esophagus which mechanically pulsates and moves the food downward. In the stomach, this is where the real work begins. If the food contains protein, hydrochloric acid (HCl), otherwise known as stomach acid, will be excreted. HCl is a barrier and first line of defense to bad guys coming in with the food (such as yeasts, bad bacteria and parasites), but more importantly, it is the fire that burns within. It is how we cook our food internally and begin the process of transforming and extracting the macro (fats, carbohydrates, proteins) and micro (vitamins, minerals) molecules from our food. Our stomach acid is SOOO important, that without it, we quickly get sick from malnourishment or invasion from outside forces.

Why is the acid in our stomach so vital? Without it we are weak in many ways:

- More susceptible to bugs from the outside.

- We cannot absorb minerals — Hello to a nation who is constantly in a panic about osteoporosis — I wonder why?!

- Can't break down our protein to absorb it properly. Protein drives detoxification, immunity and healthy neurotransmitters which mean a balanced mood and mind.

- If we are low on stomach acid, it's likely we are deficient in two key nutrients: B12 and zinc.

- Likely having acid/base balance problems in our entire body, so our stomach is not acidic, but our tissues are, where it should be the opposite. The stomach should be acidic and tissues and joints should be on the alkaline side.

Here, I'm sure you're thinking to yourself, "If there's such an epidemic of low stomach acid, then why does everyone seem to have acid reflux? Isn't that a state of having really high stomach acid? Why then are we all being prescribed Zantac and other antacid and stomach acid reducers?" This simply does not make sense.

Well here you have it, and if you know the anatomy and physiology of how the body works, specifically the stomach, it sure does make sense. Low stomach acid occurs after having a larger meal that dilutes the stomach acid. This goes along with many other physiological reasons that haven't been completely understood yet, including reducing the amount of stomach acid that is made as we age, H.Pylori infection and what is known as an acid pocket are all contributing factors to the problem[71]. To top it off, there are many concerns with regards to the treatment option using acid reducing drugs and recently, a new trend is being observed that it is not in the best interest of patients to overprescribe this class of drug[72] and here's how it all works.

The stomach has a sphincter on the top where it connects to the esophagus, for short it's known as the LES (lower esophageal sphincter). This sphincter remains open until the level of stomach acid and the amount of food is sufficient in order to break down the food.

As with all things in the D-Spot, the LES is mechanically and chemically driven, so it'll open and close depending on the stimulus. Pure genius. With a high enough level of stomach acid and not too much food, the valve will close. If you are lacking in sufficient fire in your belly, A.K.A. HCl, your LES will remain open. And if you've eaten too great a quantity of food, then you will surely lack enough of the HCl to be able to digest the food and because the quantity of food is large, your LES will remain open. This will cause the food and the little stomach acid that you may have to regurgitate upwards. This is aggravated in the evening, or if you lie down soon after a meal. It explains why people complain that they experience their symptoms worse in the evening.

In my practice this is one class of drugs we aim to get people off of, as soon as we can. They are my least favourite drugs and are known as antacids, proton pump inhibitors (PPIs) and H2 blockers. There are only a few cases where I would have patients maintain this prescription and it would only be in the case of a high cancer risk. Even then, there seems to be evidence that even on PPIs there are pathophysiological changes to the esophagus[73], not the panaceas once thought.

The biggest problem in my opinion, is losing valuable stomach acid that would prevent patients from absorbing their minerals and nutrients[74]. Minerals are so vital to a healthy body, detoxification capacity, and the immune system. As examples, zinc, selenium and magnesium. These are three major players in detox and the immune system, not to mention, they are the necessary cofactors that trigger hundreds of enzymes throughout the body, from protein manufacturing, liver detox, hormonal balance and neurotransmitter health. I wouldn't want my patients living without these keys to a healthy life.

There is another huge problem. Without the initial line of defense of the stomach, it becomes a wonderland for all types of infection. H.Pylori, as a bacteria, actually has an urease enzyme that increases the pH of the stomach, making it more basic than acidic[75]. Therefore, it becomes a hospitable zone for this bacteria and others to duplicate and infect.

The reality is that patients can get off of this prescription rather rapidly when they begin to reset their stomach acid. Ironically, most patients with gastroesophageal reflux disease, A.K.A. GERD, exhibit the lowest levels of stomach acid.

So here's where we introduce the HCl challenge. The challenge is done in order to assess the deficiency of HCl in the stomach. So the lack of fire that you've got additionally helps with resetting the stomach acid production. It seems counterintuitive that you would supplement with HCl when you are refluxing acid, but let me tell you, it works!

How To Do An HCl Challenge

You will need a bottle of HCl capsules. These typically contain hydrochloric acid and betaine and are sometimes complexed with pepsin.

Day one: One capsule before a meal
Day two: Two capsules before a meal
Day three: Three capsules before a meal

Increase your dose each day until suddenly you feel a warming sensation in the middle of your breastbone. Some people may describe it as reflux, or pressure. Once you reach that point, you then reduce at the next meal down to the dosage you were taking the day before.

Example: Say at nine capsules you felt the burn. You would then reduce down to eight capsules before every meal, for how ever long it takes to feel the sensation again. It could take two days, one week, one meal. When you feel it again, you reduce your dose again, down to seven capsules before meals.

You continue reducing the dosage in this manner until you are down to one capsule before meals. At that point, it is assumed your stomach acid would be in balance. This is a test and treatment that will likely need to be repeated. It'll be a tool in your health toolbox.

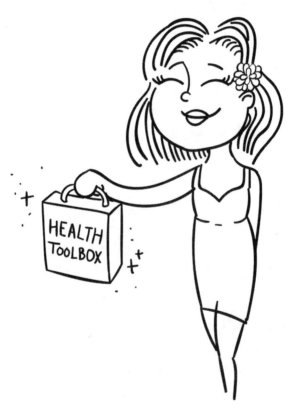

Over time, with age and complicating factors in life, your ability to have a strong fire from within can be depleted. It's a known scientific fact, that more often than not in the elderly population, they have problems most likely associated with low levels of stomach acid rather than high, and alkaline nature of reflux[76].

2. Absorption

The stomach acid has a strong pH of about 2-4. It's strong enough to rot nails. The stomach acid is meant to break down protein into smaller, more absorbable morsels for the small intestine. It also plays a key role in mineral and B12 absorption. Without proper stomach acid function, there is a tendency to have conditions associated with these deficiencies. The fire from within is specific to the breakdown of protein or possibly even bacteria, parasites and yeast (those single celled organisms). One point is that carbohydrates and fats don't absorb well in stomach acid. They begin their breakdown in the mouth and once they hit the stomach that contains HCl, the breakdown of these two macromolecules is somewhat halted.

When we are lacking proper stomach acid, this important barrier to the outside world is broken down. Bacteria, yeasts and parasites make their way down into the dungeon without much of a fight. The food you have consumed sits in the stomach, not being broken down, and is accompanied by these no good bacteria and yeasts. You have unintentionally created a haven for them and a dead zone for you.

In fact, the major issue is this dark, humid repository becomes the ideal breading zone to propagate yeasts and bad bacteria as well as becoming your very own personal fermentation factory. You may as well call your self 'Alcohol Factory (insert your full name here)'.

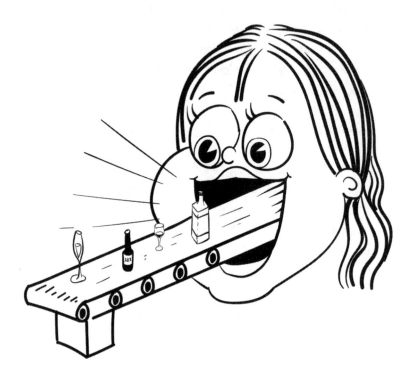

These critters are joyously devouring the food you bring them. They create alcohol as a byproduct of certain foods, which is why most people with a dysbiotic D-Spot have symptoms very similar to being hung over. What do you feel when you are hungover? You feel foggy brained, nauseated and fatigued which is the sign that your body is being overwhelmed with elevated levels of ethanol and acetyl-aldehyde breakdown in the blood[77]. The bacteria and yeast are becoming more and more numerous by the hour with this influx of fuel. When you don't have the healthiest stomach acid, there are ways to mediate this problem and most have to do with food timing and combining as well as resetting the gut (more on this later). As you can see, having a great HCl barrier is of the utmost importance.

Later we will speak about the importance of food combining, based on the body's natural physiology and supporting those principles of practice. But for now, let's continue understanding how the D-Spot delivers its deliciousness to our bodies' optimized functions.

Once the food has been churned repeatedly in the stomach, the protein has been disintegrated by the stomach acid and the carbohydrates and fats are sitting there slightly digested and waiting. Once all of the contents are the consistency of a liquid or paste, only then do the contents of the stomach begin to make their way into the duodenum.

Here, the pancreas gives them a shot of bicarbonate to continue the breakdown of fats and carbohydrates and to reduce the acidity of the stomach acid. In addition, pancreatic enzymes are further excreted to continue the breakdown of the food. The bile is then dumped from the gall bladder in the presence of fats. This helps with the first process of eliminating toxins but also improves the absorption of fats. Both the pancreas and the gall bladder use the same duct to excrete their goodness into the first part of the small intestine, the common bile duct.

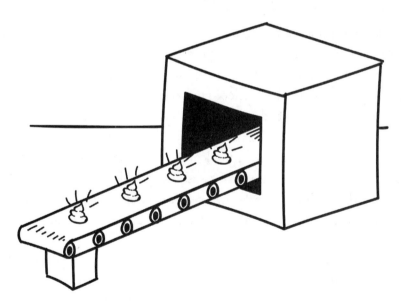

As the food makes its way down the three sections of the intestines, the duodenum is most responsible for the breakdown of food; where

carbohydrates are broken down into sugars, fats into lipids and triglycerides, and proteins into amino acids. In the jejunum and ileum, the responsibility shifts to the absorption of the smaller micromolecules and nutrients. All along the small intestine are the villi, no not villains. The villi are finger-like projections that basically "touch" the foodstuff and select what is good to absorb. The fingers feel for what they want to eat.

What helps the body to propel the food down the intestine? An important factor is the diaphragm, creating pressure gradients from inside the intestinal walls. When you take a deep belly breath this helps to propel food down the digestive tract. Most of us breathe high into our chests on a regular basis, instead of deep breathing into our bellies. If you breathe into your belly, your body would have an easier time propelling the bolus of food down the digestive tract. Later, we will learn good techniques to improve your deep breathing on a regular basis to enhance this aspect of digestion.

This key absorption area can become invaded by bad breeds of bacteria and yeast. The small intestine is tightly regulated in terms of the bacteria that it contains[78]. The bad ones often take over due to problems with our protective ability like a lack of HCl, weakened immunity and excess inflammation. These bad bugs (I like to call them conbiotics™) wreak havoc, as they are there to party and consume all the food. As they break it down it creates gas and alcohol byproducts. How do they do this? Bugs do what bugs are meant to do, they make things decay. They continue the process of breakdown and fermentation, and therefore gas production. Conbiotics™ make your small intestine a no man's land.

Now the 'bolus', which at this point is passing through the major gateway of the ileocecal valve, enters the large intestine, A.K.A. the colon. We have 5-6 meters of colon that is placed in an inverted U. This starts from the lower right side of your body up to your ribcage, then across and down the left side of your body and once again, at your left hip making an S curve called the sigmoid colon. This then descends into your rectum and anus.

The large intestine takes the food and subtracts all the water from it. The large intestine is designed with pockets called haustras. These pockets are what squeeze out what is left over that the body can't use.

The D-Spot is very efficient, nothing gets wasted and everything has a purpose. From bloating to gas, everything has its job. What's left over becomes our stools, which are bacteria and waste leftovers including fiber. Good bugs in the large intestine (probiotics) break down certain particles and actually create nutrients like B vitamins (which are water soluble and can be reabsorbed through the colon!) and certain short chained fatty aids like butyrate that are healthy for the gut[79]. The trick is this. The bacteria need to be the right kind, because the wrong type of bacteria can cause a great deal of ruckus.

3. Elimination

The large intestine is all about elimination and letting go. You must eliminate. That is its major purpose. Peristalsis that happens throughout the small and large intestine pulsates the food to where it needs to go after each step. The D-Spot is the only place in the body that has a mind of its own, as you've already learned. It can work independently of the brain, containing many of the nervous system messengers, like the endocannabinoid system[80]. That's right, regulation of intestinal motility and moving things out works with both sensation and pressure and is also regulated independently of the brain via neurotransmitters. This means that if your head was cut off, your D-Spot would still be operational. It sounds a little like a zombie apocalypse with guts walking around everywhere, digesting absorbing and eliminating.

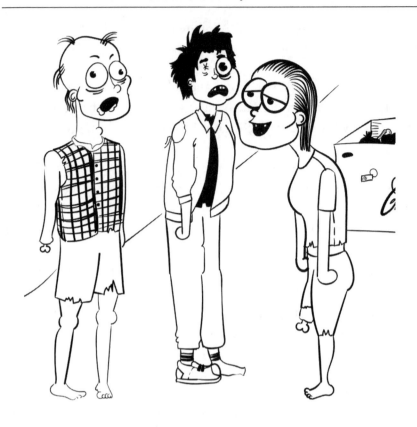

So now that you know how it works outside of the zombie apocalypse, what are the most common misconceptions about what is going on improperly with your D-Spot?

CHAPTER 4

STRESS ON THE D-SPOT

If you are good friends with Dr. Google, and you frequent the health sites, you will be familiar with names like leaky gut, Candida overgrowth or small intestine bacterial overgrowth (SIBO). These are some of the most popularized terms and are not the cause but a **side effect** of a damaged D-Spot. They are not the real problem. The real problem is usually multifactorial. What caused the gut to lose its integrity, to lose the healthy layering of mucus and length of the gut cells, to become overgrown with bad bugs and yeast and to be overtaken by toxins, both biological and chemical? What caused the gut to slowly separate itself from its friendly neighbouring cells and create gaps that allow undigested food to escape into the tissues, causing unparalleled inflammation and immune reaction? What is at the root cause of this problem? What happened here?

I'll tell you what happened, war happened. The dark side prevailed in your outside that is on your inside. The environment in your guts became so stressful, just like a war zone, that the cells are trying to get away from the badass fire from hell, the inflammation[81]. Fire only belongs in the digestive juices of the stomach; everywhere else needs peace.

When a fire rages, the body's natural response is to bring water to drown it out. What does water do? Water expands and it flows between the crevices. This also explains that when patients have a damaged D-Spot they can get very bloated, bloated to the point that they look pregnant.

The expansion is the body trying to seek balance, so it can make space to calm the fire and clean things up.

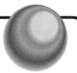

PEARL OF WISDOM

How do you know if it's more severe SIBO? A surefire symptom is bloating upon waking.

The Stress of Stress

So what about the stress that is causing this fire, this war-like reaction in the gut? The stress comes from a variety of sources. The body cannot identify the difference between stress that is physical and stress that is emotional. To the body it is all the same. Stress is stress. Stress releases the same hormones, creates the same fire, the same inflammation, no matter what the source is. Research proves that when the stress hormone cortisol is increased in the body, it degranulates mast cells that liberate histamine. Gap junctions that lose their connection are separated and the integrity of the gut is lost[82].

All stressors cause one major problem and the root cause of all disease. That one thing is inflammation[83]. It is the major culprit, yet our saving grace. This natural power is healing yet destructive. In fact, it is always discussed in the research that appropriate inflammation heals, while unregulated, it destroys[84]. It's the perfect demonstration of nature at its best. The power to heal and the power to destroy all in one.

All stressors, no matter what they are, how they look, or what they do, ultimately cause irritation and hence, inflammation. Inflammation is like a fire that burns within the body. At times, this fire is beneficial, as it destroys damaged tissue and makes way for the creation of new healthy tissue, much like in a corn field. The green leftovers of the bounty of corn get burned to feed the soil and make it rich in nutrients, prepared and ready to go for the new harvest the following year.

If the fire burns out of control and continues to propagate, it burns down fields that have not yet been harvested or it damages the farming equipment, farmhouse and barns. That fire that once helped to prepare the ground for new growth becomes a devastating inferno.

A great example of this is the relationship of chronic stress and the degeneration of the nervous system. With a little stress we have neuroplasticity. Our brain can create new networks, but with chronic long term stress we can have neurodegeneration in the form of Parkinson's and Alzheimer's disease[85].

Inflammation causes all disease, causes all dysregulation, causes all problems, from neurological decay to cancer. We need inflammation but we need to safeguard that our inflammation is healthy and does not rage like a wild forest fire. Stressors, no matter what they look like, cause inflammation, and there is a strong relationship between stress and disease[86]. The problem is the addition of multiple stressors into one system, repeatedly over time, and of long duration. This builds up a fire that is out of control.

The only way to get the fire under control is to reduce the bulk of the major stressors that are impacting the body and to quench that flame with water. Water is the universal solvent that cleans and reconnects everything. How do we know what a stressor is to our system?

We often don't. Some stressors feel good and others don't feel quite right. Sometimes we actually gravitate towards things that are not good for us. Remember those evolutionary mechanisms that were developed long before industry? We are programmed for survival, to search for high caloric food. Only, our bodies don't notice the lacking-in-nutrients part and that they may not be the best for us because they are filled with sugar, fat and salt. These cause us harm, yet we like them.

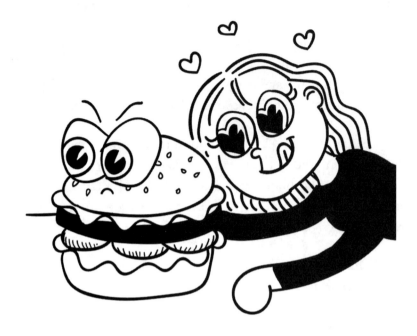

Other things like noxious scents, whether chemical or natural, are not good for us because we don't feel quite right when we inhale them. Take skunk smell, which is natural. My little Yorkie, Lola, was frolicking late one evening and she got sprayed. The smell was absolutely nauseating and made all of us in the home feel crappy. I can't even imagine how she was feeling, getting sprayed directly in her face.

When our poop smells really nasty, it isn't a good sign. In fact, healthy stools shouldn't have much of a smell at all. When there is a strong offensive scent it's a sign of bad bacteria, mucus and inflammation in the gut. Think of this - when you enter a public bathroom and you smell the lingering, awful odour of someone else's royal jewels, their bacteria is actually effecting your microbiome. And when you leave a putrid scent for someone else - you're leaving them exposed to the conbiotics™ (bad bacteria) in your system! That's why after you poop we recommend using Eau de Throne™ to freshen up the air and make it safe for the next unsuspecting victim. The organic essential oils of lavender, rosemary, clove and citrus effectively disinfect the air and neutralize embarrassing smells, they also help to calm your gut and support digestion.

The ironic thing is that a majority of the stress on our bodies comes from the outside[87] and a minor part from our inside. The greatest stressors are food, lack of food, substances we consume, foes that hijack our food, how, when and how much we eat, chemical and metabolic toxins, and our emotions. Shining light on them helps you to become aware of what is going on.

So many stressors, so little time. Here I describe the eleven top stressors that are affecting the D-Spot. Knowledge of these is powerful. So as you learn about the major stressors to the body, take note of how this is affecting your life. At the end of this chapter there is a chart with each stressor we will discuss and a scale from 1-10, 10 being a major stressor and 1 not even impacting you. As you go through each stressor, fill out the chart by rating the impact it has on your life. You will see how much of a load your body is carrying. So let's see what is stressing you out!

Stressor 1: Sugar

Remember you are **all** that you eat, so what you eat and when you eat it all has a major impact on your health. Your food can dictate what you do, your behaviours, and who you are. Now isn't that scary? Don't you think it's time for you to be more diligent about what you are feeding your beautiful temple?

Sugar is the body's most basic energy source. Everything we ingest has the ability to become sugar. If that is the case, it's hard to believe that something like this can lead us astray.

Simply put, it's all about moderation. Too much sugar and it makes your body go crazy. Sugar resembles the body's stress hormone and that's why they call it a glucocorticoid. No matter where the sugar comes from, sugar looks like sugar. When we get stressed, the hormone cortisol gets pumped out and sugar is released. The reason being is to feed your muscles in the case where you need to run away from a predator. Yes that's right, run away from a predator. Most of us no longer encounter the normal four legged predators from the past.

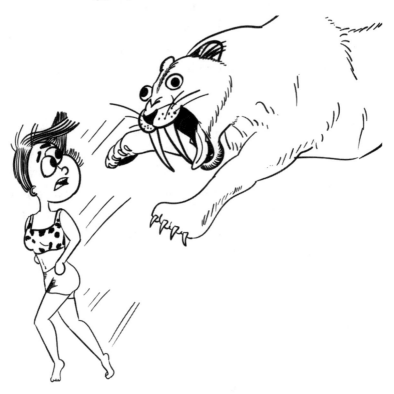

There is a new type of predator on the scene and they're much nicer to look at. Say hello to desserts, large carbohydrate boasting meals, alcoholic beverages and dessert-like coffee drinks from the coffee shop on the corner. These predators all sneak into our daily practices for the simple reason that they are intertwined into our cultural and social habits and they taste really, really good.

In nature, sugar is not found on its own, it is combined with fiber and nutrients and in that state, the sugar is healthy. It also isn't necessarily found all year long. Sugar is found mostly at the end of summer, when all of the fruits ripen. In tropical countries, all fruits have their season and they should be eaten at that time. We have a special evolutionary sweet tooth that makes us love sugary, sweet things, because the ripening of fruits signalled the coming of winter, which meant less fresh bounty and the possibility of scarcity and starvation. Back in the day, we used to have to hibernate.

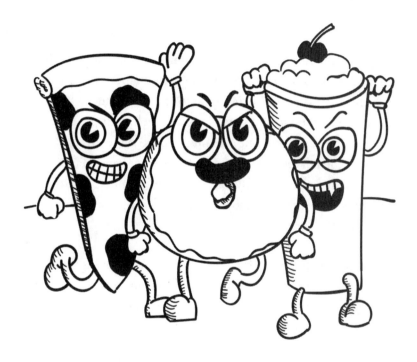

Now we feed our evolutionary sweet tooth all of the time, with no breaks. The result is our bodies' own natural receptors that detect sugar and bring it into the cell, are revolting. They shut down due to the high levels of sugar flowing through our bodies and we have what is called metabolic syndrome that is rooted in insulin resistance[88], the precursor to Type II diabetes. The result is we don't feel well. In fact, we feel starved in a land of plenty. This is the reality that is linked to our present day epidemic and leading causes of death by cardiovascular disease[89] and cancer[90]. In fact, high levels of blood sugar, which is known as hyperglycemia, can negatively impact treatments and outcomes of cancer patients[91].

At their root is elevated blood glucose levels and insulin resistance. In fact, at the root of most disease is an elevated sugar level, because sugar is a stressor and stressors cause inflammation, and inflammation is linked to every disease that affects man! You can see how important it is to reduce the blood sugar level.

The damage that sugar can do is major. It can affect the small little blood vessels and damage them to the point that they can't receive blood and oxygen. This is one of the reasons why diabetics can lose limbs, because they literally lose their supply of nourishment. The same can happen to the nerves, losing sensations and feeling in the limbs, losing eyesight, losing taste, hearing, mental acuity, basically any function governed by the nerves. The sugar itself does not cause damage but it's something called advanced glycolysation end products (AGE's). These are basically free radicals made of sugar that attack the tissues, via inflammation[92].

High fructose corn syrup (HFCS) is worth mentioning here, as it is produced from corn, but is in epidemic levels in most of our foods. It makes up approximately 40% of caloric sweeteners used in the United States today[93]. You can find HFCS in most processed foods from salad dressings to TV dinners. A major problem with HFCS is that it spikes the blood sugar when the average American consumes 50g per day but research also shows that it contains levels of mercury[94]. So it doubly affects our bodies in a negative way. Artificial maple syrups are made of HFCS. To me, if you are going to eat maple syrup it may as well be the good stuff that actually has health promoting aspects like being chock full of minerals. On the scale at the end of this chapter, fill in your sugar stress from 1 to 10.

Stressor 2: Alcohol (Liquid Sugar)

We have developed a cultural practice of using alcohol as a relaxing agent but also as a social tool. Many of us who feel stressed or tense use this as an excuse to indulge in the liquid love. It calms us down, but at the same time disrupts our sleep and wake cycle[95]. A little bit is good but too much is hazardous for your health.

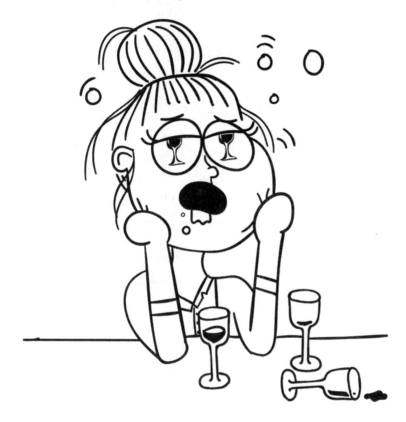

We all know that too much alcohol can damage our livers, and for some of us, an addiction that is hard to break. However, the dangers of alcohol go beyond that in terms of your D-Spot health. Alcohol is a product of fermentation and as such, fermentation products can irritate an unhealthy D-Spot[96].

Fermented foods create a natural neurotransmitter and chemical messenger known as histamine[97]. This molecule, you have likely heard of, is associated with the allergic response and symptoms such as a runny nose, watery eyes, closing of the throat, hives or a rash you would get from exposure to poison ivy. Histamine causes a lot of inflammation and irritation and it's a tool that the body uses to heal. It creates inflammation to bring the good blood cells to the area to do the clean up.

In a damaged D-Spot, the effect of too much histamine means big problems. You can imagine that it would create a similar inflammatory rash in the intestines as poison ivy does to the skin. Worse, it's the culprit that causes the tight gap junctions to separate, making your gut leaky. Since the skin, brain and gut have links that connect them to embryonic tissue, they respond similarly to different insults. The interesting thing is that people who have neurological inflammation, such as children on the autism spectrum, have conditions associated with high levels of mast cell degranulation and hence, histamine in the brain[98]. There is a connection known as the gut-brain axis which makes this pattern repeat in the gut[99].

I look at histamine like little army men with machine guns. When they come into play, they just shoot to kill everything with no regard whether it is friend or foe.

They are a form of communication in the system, albeit, they haven't learned the skill of peaceful discussion[100].

The other issue with alcohol is that it is liquid sugar, so it will feed a dysbiotic D-Spot.

This, in terms of the D-Spot, is the other huge problem. Alcohol can really take a toll on your D-Spot and is a stressor best avoided if you're having digestive symptoms. Add your alcohol stress on a scale of 1-10 at the end of this chapter.

Stressor 3: Processed Foods

What makes food, food? Food is a combination of macromolecules (protein, fat & sugars) designed in perfect combination by nature. They provide us with calories, which in turn, provide us with micromolecules such as vitamins and minerals. These foods are easy to digest and give our body what it needs. Usually foods have a shelf life and break down over time with exposure to air and heat. Food should also look like it does in nature. Broccoli shouldn't look like a cabbage and watermelon should have seeds. Food is simply food, it tastes good and benefits the body.

When we mess with mother nature, as the nutrition engineers and food manufacturers do, we usually end up causing stress to natural systems in one way, shape or form.

Food that has been over processed and highly packaged isn't recognized by the body because it does not exist in nature. Our bodies have evolved to absorb food in its natural state, slightly modified by cooking with fire or by being fermented, only as nature would have it.

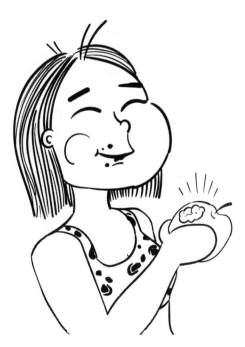

When over processed by taking the germ out of the wheat or the lactose out of the milk, suddenly you have this foreign molecule that the body has no clue how to use. The food may have become more aesthetically attractive but it serves us no benefit, like white bread. It may be easier to digest such as the case with lactose-free milk, but did you ever think there may be a reason why you shouldn't ingest it?

Processing to package it for convenience adds heat. Heat depletes nutrients, so in each step of the process, the more heated a food stuff is, the more it is depleted in nourishment. They heat it as it's being packaged as a form of preservation and then once again, you nuke it to warm it up so you can eat it. This equals devitalized food.

Those nutritional scientists add in ingredients that prevent natural decay. They achieve this by adding ingredients, such as excess high fructose corn syrup (HFCS), sodium, potassium sorbate, calcium EDTA and other preservatives. Their goal is to prevent what is natural; for the food to rot, and for bacteria to grow. Once again we can't recognize these food ingredients, except the HFCS and sodium which will actually make the food more enjoyable for you, hooking you in the process. Nature decays; it's not natural to stay preserved.

Some foods that have been manipulated are within their natural state. For example, genetically modified organisms (GMOs). Seedless tomatoes and watermelons are not the norm and neither is an apple the size of a melon nor broccoli that is purple. These variations in genetics are completely out of sync with what nature intended. So much so, that the European Union has outright banned GMO foods coming into the country.

With good reasons, many of these GMO foods are resistant to the most commonly used herbicide, glyphosate (Round-up). They have been developed to not be damaged when they are sprayed. The big issue now is that this pesticide is potentially toxic at lower than normal levels[101].

The GMO and Round-up ready plants grow and are resistant, which makes them attractive to farmers, but they bio-accumulate the pesticides more than conventional and organic produce[102]. Interesting to note, the organic produce is more resilient to the chemical impact, however, it still has accumulation.

In a 2 year study on rats, this herbicide and the Round-up tolerant GMO corn caused serious health effects across the entire body, including an increase in earlier death in the female subjects along with large mammary tumours, liver issues in males, kidney and pituitary pathologies across both sexes. This herbicide effect is widespread to what was once thought as only an endocrine or neurological disruptor. More research needs to be done but the writing is on the wall. It's not as nature intended, so it has a negative effect on our nature[103].

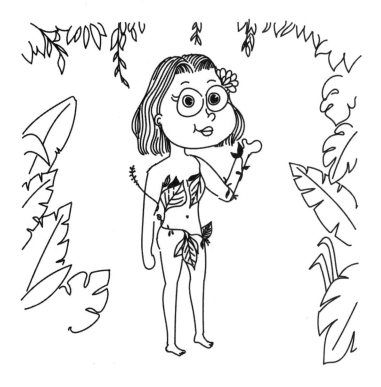

Certain genetic traits, specifically people that have a homozygous PON 1 gene, like myself, are extremely sensitive to exposure with this herbicide. Since glyphosate is a neurological toxicant, my body, to protect itself, increases estrogen, so I in turn get these splotches of darkened skin called melasma, the marks of pregnancy.

It is discussed that glyphosate also has an anti-microbial effect on the bugs of the gut[104]. It has the potential to disrupt the natural microbiota, not only of the ruminants, but also of the humans who are consuming food that has been sprayed or that contains the herbicide due to cross contamination. The highly pathogenic bacteria such as Clostridium and Salmonella seem to be highly resistant to glyphosate, whereas the beneficial bacteria such as Bifido spp. and Lactobacillis spp. are moderately to highly susceptible to this chemical. This leaves us with pathogenic strains becoming stronger, and healthier strains losing their stance. That is very dangerous for the D-Spot in the longterm.

Being the most widespread and commonly used herbicide in the USA since its launch in 1974, over 1.6 billion kg of glyphosate has been sprayed. This has significantly polluted our environment and harmed our eco-systems. In 1996 there was a staggering increase in the amount that was and continues to be sprayed on crops worldwide. It's a force to be reckoned with that has infiltrated every aspect of our lives, our water supply and our food supply, including all crops and our livestock, and has completely disrupted how we farm[105].

If you thought we were in the homestretch, think again. A weird fact is that many processed foods have surprise ingredients, such as aluminum. This is a toxic metal that is found to be higher in processed foods than unprocessed[106]. Basically, this serves to prove the point that you really don't know what you are getting with over processed and packaged foods. Be wary!

The jury is out, natural is the way to go if you want to cause less stress to the system. Natural is simply better.

As you begin to become aware of these situations and "buy-cott" the packaged and processed foods, changes begin to happen. Make your vote with your dollar. It's what counts for your health. Don't forget to rate your processed foods stress at the end of the chapter!

Stressor 4: Caffeine

Every time I bring this one up, people always look at me and say, "No, don't take my coffee away!" Then they pipe up, "Dr. Oz says it's good for me!" True, there are components of coffee, such as chlorogenic acid, that are known to have beneficial effects for the D-Spot by helping to improve the amount of Bifido bacteria that colonize the gut[107]. Bifido bacteria is important because it is a source of butyric acid that heals the D-Spot. You got me! That part of coffee is healthy.

I'm not saying that coffee is overall bad for you, but remember our goal. Reduce the load of overall stress on the system. Caffeine, in its many forms - coffee, tea, soda pop and energy drinks is a stressor because it is an irritant to the nervous system. It irritates the D-Spot, as it's an area with highly neurologically active tissues. Research shows that when caffeine is consumed on its own it accentuates the physiological stress response.

In utero, caffeine can create health problems long term for the infant. Because caffeine is an adenosine receptor antagonist, it can stimulate heart and metabolic output problems as well as epigenetic changes when consumed while pregnant[108]. This action, as an adenosine receptor antagonist, is what exerts its affect over the nervous system, causing symptoms of anxiety, including tremors, insomnia and digestive symptoms like nausea and diarrhea[109].

Other issues with caffeine are that it enhances insulin resistance[110] and when combined with sugar, gives a synergistic effect that further perturbs insulin resistance[111]. It is possibly linked to rheumatoid arthritis and Type 1 Diabetes, both classified as autoimmune conditions[112] [113] where the immune system attacks its own tissues. Evidence suggests that individuals with allergies, upon caffeine intake, alter their gut bacteria, potentially complicating their condition[114].

When caffeine is taken with L-theanine, a calming agent found in green tea, they cancel each other out[115]. The anxiety producing effect of caffeine and the relaxing effect of theanine negate each other. This is one of the reasons why green tea is one beverage that is recommended when healing the D-Spot, and especially for those wanting to wean off of their favourite drink, coffee, which has been known to be as addictive as opiates[116].

Interesting to note, the negative caffeine effect is dose dependant. Too much is no good, and a little is just right[117]. The D-Spot needs calmness and relaxation to feel good and operate efficiently. Giving the body a literal jolt of caffeine just stresses your system and that's not our goal. Reduce the stress. Now rate yours in this category, it may be your highest one yet!

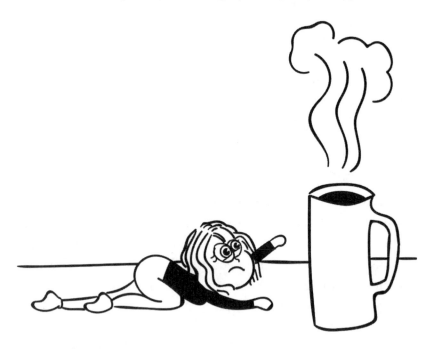

Stressor 5: Starvation

The ultimate stress is starvation. It's rare in this day and age that we deal with true starvation; one that is forced upon us. There is always food at our disposal, Big Mac here, Whopper there, Super Size Me anywhere.

At any given moment we can get calories. The only problem is that food is so much more than just calories.

Calories don't feed our souls. They feed our waist lines and the inflammation in our D-Spots. Most of us are starving in a land of plenty. Food is nourishment which means that it needs to be chock full of vitamins, minerals and nutrients if it is going to serve us, not just calories. Calories must count. Otherwise we are basically starving and we can't escape the calories either. Hence the obesity epidemic.

Take the use of artificial sweeteners to satisfy our taste buds and avoid calories in the hopes of staying slim. This results in an altering of our metabolism and insulin responses, thwarting our evolutionary sweet taste perception and our gut bugs working against us, making us want, crave and eat more food[118] [119]!

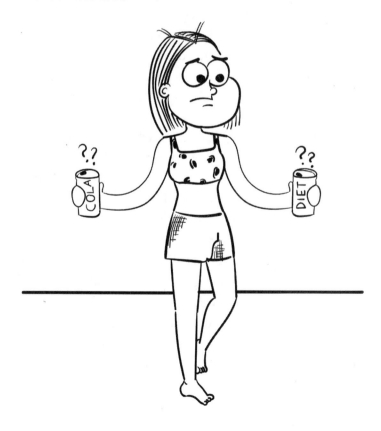

Playing God with our responses to sugar has created the perfect environment for us to easily "catch" metabolic syndrome or Type II Diabetes. Our bodies have evolved from an evolutionary perspective to be very precocious about using our sugar during periods of starvation. There are multiple ways that the body can survive.

The all-mighty glucose (A.K.A. sugar) can be made from protein, or ketones can be made from fat. Glucose is required for cells without mitochondria to live, like red blood cells. Most of the body and brain can survive on ketones. This preservation of glucose for the cells that need it, is embedded into our DNA, a protective mechanism that sets us up for metabolic derangement[120].

When stress is high in the system, as in long term starvation, the body breaks down essential amino acids in the muscles. Whereas in non-stressed states, it will selectively use non-essential amino acids; glutamine, alanine, glycine and (hydroxy)proline. Even if the stress persists and if re-feeding begins, the breakdown of muscle continues[121] in the same manner. Wasting of the essential amino acids will only stop once the stress stops. Then the building of muscle can restart.

Starving is either self inflicted or other imposed. Some slave to fit into society to what is expected to be the norm for the female or male body. Eating disorders such as anorexia and bulimia have the same effect as other imposed starvations. Survivors of the holocaust experienced severe other imposed starvation and the repercussions are all the same. In chronically starved patients, it is noted that the cellular metabolism of the fat free mass is greatly reduced. This preservation mechanism, as well as being a key metabolic derangement in our bodies, can exist with us for the longterm, post chronic stress of starvation[122]. This starvation not only impacts the survivors but the future generations as well[123].

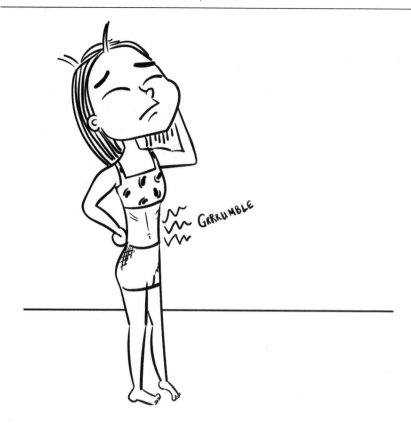

What are the direct systemic effects of not having good quality food or of choosing to not feed your body? It deranges your metabolism and ultimately causes stress. It sets you up to have inflammation, insulin resistance (A.K.A. metabolic syndrome) and a D-Spot that is damaged. Starving is stressful.

Stressor 6: Food Sensitivities

Healthy food, or so you think, may be your poison.

When I explain to people about food sensitivities, I give them my life story which explains it all. I was very unhealthy when I was in my early 20s but I had started to have a sort of health revolution once I hit my mid to late 20s. I visited multiple naturopaths to get me on my "natural path" (pun intended). So with each naturopath, I would embark on a different, yet similar type of detox/cleanse diet to help myself feel better. The only problem was that every time I would start one of these diets, I would gradually feel sicker and sicker and more bloated and lethargic. I really started to think something was truly wrong with me, each naturopath would say, "It's just part of the healing reaction", so I would keep on, eventually feeling so badly that I would have no choice but to give up.

What a lesson! Oh, Sh*t! I couldn't understand. Here I am, eating the healthiest of foods, rice, broccoli, kale, almonds, turmeric… I'm not even touching the big bad food allergens, and I feel like total sh*t! There is something so wrong with me. I am doomed! Being determined to feel better, I kept on trying, without results. Then finally, when I was in school to become a naturopath, as most of us do in order to help heal ourselves, I asked one of my mentors to run my food sensitivity panel. I had not been offered that by the other naturopaths so I figured, "Hey, I may as well try it. At $600 a pop as a starving student, what have I got to lose?"

Then when I received my results, my entire thought paradigm shifted in terms of food sensitivities. I become 100% enlightened. Worth every penny! My sensitivities were rice, kale, almonds and turmeric. These were all of the foods on a detox diet that I was trying to over consume in an effort to get healthy. What's healthy for one may not be your personal panacea of health. I encourage all of my patients to run their food sensitivity testing as it makes their treatment so much easier. Check out the resource page at the back of this book for a link to a lab that I use and trust where you can get food sensitivity testing done.

Your D-Spot is exposed to food daily and if you're eating something that you are not meant to eat, it's a major block to healing.

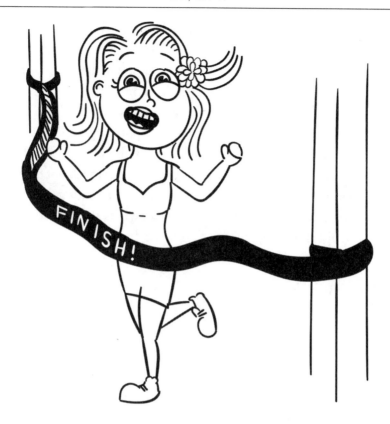

Allergies, sensitivities and intolerances are not all created equally. People are always asking, "I have an allergy to peanut, so what's the difference between that and a sensitivity or intolerance?" Or they say, "Oh, my doctor already tested for allergies and I don't have any." Well I always inquire which test they did, because every test, tests for something different.

Allergies

Allergies are most commonly understood as the anaphylactic type and can be life threatening. They affect 4-7% of pre school children[124], and the prevalence for food allergy in Europe is approximately 0.1-6%[125]. The most common reaction is to cow's milk, egg, peanut, tree nuts, wheat, soy, shellfish and finned fish.

The immediate response is the throat closes and breathing becomes laboured and difficult. There is also a delayed allergic response that can manifest up to 48 hours later such as seasonal allergies, dust, cat, dog or poison ivy. Most of these include runny watery eyes, sniffles and difficulty breathing. A skin rash may be present as well. An allergy which I find is quite peculiar, that has been popping up in practice quite often, is a sensitivity to hot and cold. That is the ultimate in allergic responses. It is a sign that our immune system is very much out of whack and even a slight stimulus such as temperature can make it go wild. The test that medical doctors typically run is known as the scratch test, as it shows the IgE immune mediated response[126].

Sensitivities

Sensitivities are immediate up to 72 hours later, a delayed reaction response. They manifest differently in all types of body systems, are mediated by IgG and generally triggered by food. In conventional medical circles, they are often referred to as "delayed-onset non-IgE-mediated manifestation of food allergy[127]". Naturopaths often classify these as food sensitivities. Since they don't only show up in the gut and they can present themselves all over the body, it can be hard to detect what is causing what. The gold standard elimination diet is tedious and difficult. Patients lose their willpower and most opt in to do food sensitivity testing in order to simplify their lives. My experience has been that very few people are the same. There are some commonalities that pop up in the testing, such as certain nuts and legumes. However, most people have one or two sensitivities that are very random. When trying to heal the gut, if those are not identified it could be their barrier to cure. Check out the resource page at the back of the book for a link to lab testing that I use and trust.

Intolerances

Intolerances are typically due to a lack of enzymes or inability to digest and absorb a food[128]. A common intolerance includes lactose, where you cannot break down the sugar found in milk. Symptoms are typically diarrhea and disturbing gas. Other intolerances include an inability to properly digest different food groups together. This was first popularized by the Carroll Food Intolerance Method and the health book Fit for Life by Marilyn and Harvey Diamond, where certain proteins are not combined with certain carbohydrates. An example of this is rice and protein. Because of the way the digestive track works, most carbohydrates, especially those of the starchy variety, do not digest well with protein. Protein and greens in general do digest well together. When you make a combination of hard to digest foods, it can upset your D-Spot significantly.

Got Glue?

My best and favourite example of this is how glue is made. Glue is an example of an intolerance of combining certain foods together (they also happen to highlight the most important food sensitivities and allergies that people deal with). White school glue, if you didn't know, is actually edible. It's made with milk, sugar and flour and then the ingredient that is the pièce de résistance is vinegar[129]. This combination is basically exactly what happens in your belly, when you combine bread (flour) with cheese (dairy/milk) and you swallow it down into your stomach that contains your stomach acid (like vinegar because it's acidic!). Guess what, you've got glue in your belly!

So Imagine what your gut is like, if you are consuming glue. Remember the villi, the finger like projections in the small intestine? They get stuck together and reduce your ability to properly digest your food! In addition, because the carbohydrates and protein don't digest well together, you get this glue moving all along your digestive tract. Worse still, if you look at typical eating patterns. Most meals, for instance breakfast, supposedly the most important meal of the day, is typically a combination of flour (cereal) and milk, and even worse if you add egg, which is used as a strong binder in baking. So here are most of us and our children starting our day off by gluing up our guts!

The ultimate end problem with allergies, sensitivities and intolerances is that they cause stress and aggravation to your divine D-Spot. If you are trying to heal your D-Spot, it will be an uphill battle if you haven't addressed these issues. For every two steps forward, you will move three steps backward. It's important to remove all the irritants in order to have healing.

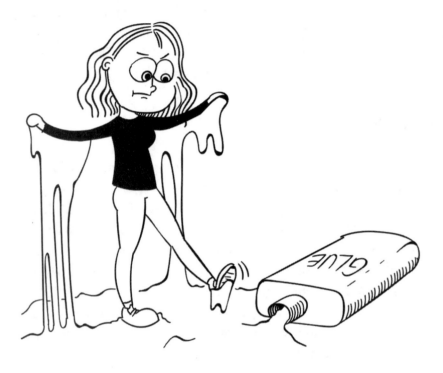

Don't be fooled into thinking that your allergies, sensitivities and intolerances have disappeared. Patients would say, "I used to have a problem with milk, but it doesn't bother me anymore". I've heard this many times. Unfortunately, people are mistaken. Unless you've healed your gut, allergies, sensitivities and intolerances never disappear, they just transform, go deeper or you become numb to them.

As they go deeper, they start to bother other aspects of your body such as long term ongoing joint pain or depression. The problem has just created inflammation in a different tissue[130].

On the other hand, because you are putting so much of the allergen into your system, your body reduces the response to it. Your body basically says, "Hey, well if you're not going to listen to me, why should I bother making noise?" It then simply knocks out the immune system reaction, which leaves you weak against other invaders and cancer.

The only thing that can go away is your degree of sensitivity. Many foods are either a true sensitivity or they may be a sensitivity caused by overexposure. For me, as an example, rice was one of my sensitivities. Now, if you haven't figured it out already, I'm Spanish. I grew up and consumed a boatload of rice in my lifetime. It is one of my favourite foods, hands down. Paella anyone?

For me, it became a sensitivity because I just plain overdid it. Once I stopped consuming it for a period of over one year, I would have it here and there but never religiously. On my follow-up food sensitivity testing, it wasn't a true sensitivity anymore. As long as I moderate the consumption of rice, all is well. If I overdo it, I will feel it! This I have seen replicated in many patients numerous times. The key is that the reduction of exposure of the food sensitivity needs to take place over at least one year, and while you are generally working on health practices that heal your D-Spot. More on this important subject later. Rate your food sensitivity stress on a scale of 1-10.

Stressor 7: Emotion

The D-Spot is divine and delightful because it is one of the ways through which we feel emotion. Therefore, it is highly susceptible to being "distraught" when the emotional climate of our lives is not balanced. Some say that The D-Spot feels, as discussed before, as it is the centre of our intuition and excitement. It's our area from which we are nourished, and if we can't nourish ourselves because we are reactive to everything, perhaps we could also be lacking nourishment from those who love us. Our D-Spot is so interconnected to the stress we feel that it actually has a condition named after it for a stressful bowel. That condition is irritable bowel syndrome (IBS) for those of you who don't know.

I am one of those persons, as is my father, who deals with IBS. I feel stress and anxiety, good and bad, all in my D-Spot. It's why, as a naturopathic doctor, my mission is to help people reset their D-Spot, to live their lives well because a damaged spot is detrimental to your ultimate health goal and having an exceptional quality of life. Let me tell you that I know where every toilet is. Why? Because stressors for me go directly to my D-Spot. The more sensitive you are, and if you are sensitive like me, the more that you feel it. You may either have IBS that is classically a diarrhea type, or the type that is predominantly constipation, or the type that moves into both constipation and diarrhea. I am fortunate to have the latter.

I am a very sensitive person. I feel all the pain and emotions in my stomach and when I am dealt an excessive amount of stress, my D-Spot reacts appropriately in order to protect my body. It says, "Oh Sh*t, I don't feel good right now, I'm not being nourished. Perhaps it is something you ate? Perhaps it's how you are feeling? Perhaps there is some toxin that came from the outside that is irritating me, or just the thought of it? AGGGHH, I don't know. The best thing to do is EVACUATE!" 'Swoosh' go the bowels. It is a self protective mechanism to eliminate when under stress. For those who are sensitive, there is hope. The key is to look at all the stressors, and sometimes you need to go very deep to figure out what is triggering your D-Spot.

You can't run away from your emotions. They affect you. They both nourish or deprive your body and soul. You can learn to work with your emotions and reduce how you perceive stressors. It is important to learn relaxing techniques and health practices that significantly reduce the amount of cortisol (the stress hormone) that is flying through your body (hello castor oil packs!). When you are healing the gut, you must also address the soul and your stress. The two are intertwined and mutually dependent on each other. The D-Spot, being the second brain, can feel. It's part of what allows it to "feel" your food, "feel" for an intruder, to "feel" that you are not feeling quite right. It is the temperature gauge of your emotions, and you don't want it on high heat all of the time.

Stress is one of the most important factors in disease. Emotional stress cannot be denied. Granted, there are times when managing your emotional stress may be difficult (the passing of a loved one as an example). You need to work to lift yourself from where you are at, focus on what you have and be grateful. Practising health can greatly reduce your stress. If that's the best you can do, then that is great. Just don't sit there and do nothing, unless you are meditating... And then hey, you are on the right track.

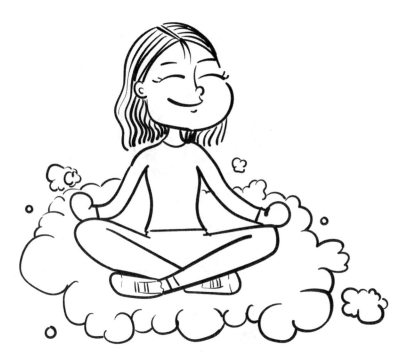

There has been so much research done on the benefits of meditating. Active focus on calm and relaxation takes you internally and connects you to who you are and to all of life. It is an important practice, even if you do it for simply just five minutes per day. Everyone needs to start somewhere. Castor oil packs can be an excellent complement to meditative practice - more on this later.

Honour your emotions. Don't disregard the triggers from your past that are affecting you today. To work through them, all that needs to be done is to sit with them and to feel them. When suppressed and pushed into the shadows, they become an irritant that affects your D-Spot.

Emotionally, the D-Spot and specifically the large intestine, is known for its ability to let go. You may have a tendency of holding onto things and not working through them. If you hoard from both a physical and emotional level, you likely have issues with constipation. Your body tends to freeze and it slows down its activity to protect you.

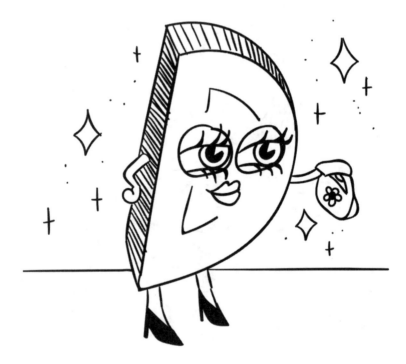

You can't deny it, the D-Spot has DRAMA and is likely a bit of a diva. As long as you know what you are working with, you can make changes that will help to make your emotional centre well balanced. Rate your emotional stress in the chart at the end of this chapter.

Stressor 8: Dysbiotic D-Spot - Yeast, Bacteria and Parasites

Where there is life, there are bugs. Where there is decay, there are bugs. By bugs, I mean bacteria, yeast and parasites. The bugs are either opportunistic, taking advantage of a host to propagate, or they are symbiotic, actually working together for the greater good to push the system forward. There is no living thing that does not co-exist with bugs. None. In one way, shape or form, we need them to survive.

For humans, certain strains of bacteria, such as lactobacillus acidophilus and bifidobacteria in the large intestine, actually produce vitamins for us. Some also help us to further break down our food, helping in the digestion process and healing the gut. They do our body good and are necessary for our lives. We feed them and they feed us. We have been working like a team for quite some time. A big job of the good gut bacteria like L. Acidophilus, is to keep the gut in check - the healthy bacteria high and bad bacteria and yeast, low[131]. They defend their environment and that means defending you. Their neck is in it as much as it is for you.

Many people think, "Ah, here, let's take this probiotic which contains billions of bacteria and multiple different strains" (sometimes up to 15 strains). The only issue is that each strain of bacteria has a different action[132]. This is not common knowledge, but it's knowledge that needs to spread, just like a bacterial infection! There are strains of bacteria that may or may not be beneficial for you depending on your state of health. As an example, multi-strain probiotics are effective in gastrointestinal conditions and some strains show no effect when placed alone, namely L. Acidophillus, L. Plantarum, and B. Infantis[133]. Keep in mind this is only the results of one meta-analysis and that things are constantly changing.

Then there are the bacteria like Clostridium difficile (C. difficile), that are downright mean and nasty. The mere mention of this bacteria sends hospital staff running to begin emergency evacuation. These bacteria are aggressive and wreck havoc in the intestine, causing major diarrhea and can even cause death. It's no different than cholera caused by the strain of bacteria Vibrio cholerae (V. cholerae), or a more common one, E. coli. Our food supply is being invaded more and more by the bad strains. It's a regular occurrence that some food is being recalled for Listeria contamination[134]. We call these bad bugs conbiotics™, because they are like con artists, using up all of our vital resources and claiming the 'turf' of our guts as their own.

We have other bugs that are not so nice and prey on our resources, depleting us of nutrients, like parasites. Parasites require a host, and from the host they extract nutrients and deplete us. They cause all types of uncomfortable symptoms and we can become malnourished, weak and less likely to fight them off.

Then there are the yeasts. Research is still in its infancy as to what is known about the mycobiome. However, the connection is clear that it has an impact on our health[135]. A very common yeast, that has a bad rap in natural health circles is Candida albicans. We all have Candida in our system. Normally, when we are well behaved, eating a nice balanced diet, not overdoing it on processed foods, sugar or alcohol, our good bacteria will keep our Candida levels in check. The good bacteria safeguard our gut environment so there is no propagation of the bad guys. The only issue is when you start abusing your D-Spot or if it is already damaged.

Is it a war down there? It definitely can be. There are many reasons the D-Spot has become dysbiotic and is dysfunctioning.

1. **Stomach acid is sub-optimal**. As we discussed before, it's nature's selective barrier as to what gets in and what does not. When you are lacking your true stomach fire, you allow the bad gut bugs in with the food that you eat. This sets up a bug replication and formation super party. The D-Spot is the ideal

place, dark and humid, for the bugs to propagate. Naturally, we do have bugs in our D-Spot but they find themselves in highest concentration in the large intestine. There are a few selective strains in the small intestine, the duodenum, jejenum and ileum. Your stomach acid dictates who's invited to the party. A great example of this is a stomach infected with H.Pylori. This nasty bug actually releases a urease that turns off your stomach acid producing cells and with it, their bactericidal activity[136]. So it makes it easy for H.pylori to survive along with many friends that don't belong in your D-Spot.

2. **Food is meant to decay.** Wherever there is food, you will find natural decay and with it, bacteria and yeast. The more decay there is, the more yeast and bacteria. One simple way of reducing the amount of unhealthy yeast and bacteria that come into your body is to reduce the amount of time that you store your food, and to try and consume fresh food. That's why, if something is rotting, you should be throwing it away in lieu of keeping it for future use.

3. **History of taking antibiotics and antifungals.** If you have a history of taking many rounds of antibiotics, such as children who've taken repetitive rounds due to ear infections, or teenagers due to acne, or middle aged women due to yeast or urinary tract infections[137]... mind my message here. If you ever take antibiotics or antifungals, please ensure that you are taking a HIGH QUALITY probiotic in between doses to avoid getting secondary infections[138]. Yogurt is NOT enough[139]. It is also full of sugar that can feed the conbiotics™. Ideally, take a probiotic that is coated, to ensure it enters the body and gets deep into the gut, or take your probiotics on an empty stomach with an alkalinizing agent on waking and before bed.

4. **When you were only a bun in the oven!** Many factors affect the initial populating by bugs in your D-Spot. From prenatal

to post delivery, environmental and lifestyle factors have a profound effect on the microbiota and on immunoregulation during early life[140]. If you are born via caesarean section instead of being born via the vagina, you get your first inoculation of bugs from the hospital's environment. That can be chock full of not very good stuff! In addition, if your mother took antibiotics or other immune-disrupting drugs while pregnant it will effect the population of bugs in your developing D-Spot. These two factors increase your chances of having eczema as a child, a condition characteristic of a damaged microbiome and D-Spot[141]. Our body, bugs and D-Spot learn early on what they want and crave.

5. **Spending time with sick people.** The greater frequency and amount of time that you're around people that are sick, the higher likelihood of you having unhealthy gut flora. Hospitals and health care workers have to be very cautious to prevent getting a nosocomial infection, A.K.A. hospital acquired infection. Staying clean and being accountable are why systems are installed such as Hand Hygiene Monitoring programs[142] to keep workers free from infection or from spreading it. This helps but it doesn't completely solve the problem, as bacteria and yeast are everywhere on the skin, you simply cannot run or hide!

6. **You are a product of your environment.** An environment that is damp, moist and has the possibility of mold or bacteria growth, will be reflected in your health. It will make your internal environment more hospitable to infection with yeast and bacteria as they thrive within this environment. Research proves that people living in these environments are more susceptible to rhinitis infections[143]. If everyone in your home is ill with inflictions such as yeast overgrowth, sinus congestion and constant lung infections, you need to begin to look at your environment as a source of the weakness in your microbiome and hence your immunity.

7. **Your mouth is a bacterial DANGER ZONE.** Imagine that the mouth is a cesspool for bacteria, with over 700 species cohabiting. The ecology of the mouth is gently balanced by our oral hygiene, the foods we eat, and the amount of dental work we have had. The concept of a bacterial biofilm that needs to be regularly removed to protect one's health from infectious bacteria is important. The biofilm is the causative factor in carries, tooth decay, periodontal diseases and worse infectious diseases in other parts of the body[144]. Candida biofilms are common in secondary and persistent root canal infections[145] and root canals have been suspected, since the early 1900s, to be a constant source of endotoxins for the body[146], known as foci or focal infection. Unfortunately, on many occasions, this has been disputed by conventional medicine, but once again it comes to the forefront of science as having elements of truth[147]. Oil pulling is the ancient Ayurvedic practice of swishing oil in the mouth to reduce bad bacteria and balance the microbiome. It is commonly done with coconut oil, swishing for about 20 minutes, but even more effective is doing this with castor oil. Castor oil has been shown to be extremely effective in periodontal medicine for breaking down biofilm[148 149 150], and you only need to swish for two minutes for the benefit. There are strong links to the health of your mouth and the health of your body. After all, the D-Spot microbiome begins in the mouth, as on top, so down below.

8. **Stress is always at fault.** Stress is always at fault because it is the root cause of all disease, including overgrowth of bad bugs within the gut. Stress makes your gut susceptible to infection because it weakens the natural barrier that keeps you healthy. These stressors come from food components such as oxalates or lectins that all create irritation in the gut or other "stressful factors". From the stomach acid to the tight junctions of the cells that line the D-Spot, they all become weak with stress. The more stressed your system is, the higher likelihood of

having infectious bacteria, yeasts and parasites[151]. Like attracts like. When you are healthy, happy and stress-free, you attract healthy and unstressed bacteria. When your system is stressed you attract negative stressed bugs. My first go-to in helping with stress are my nightly castor oil packs, which also create the perfect environment to get a great night's sleep.

9. **The masked mycotoxins.** Common cereal crops, legumes, nuts, and fruits are a source of a poison, something known as a masked mycotoxin. These masked mycotoxins are produced during the growth, post harvest in storage, and during transport of these crops. They are secondary fungal metabolites. You may have heard of aflatoxins, which are found on peanuts. Their claim to fame is that they are a carcinogenic compound, thus promoting cancer, specifically liver[152]. Initially, the thought was that these components of food weren't digested in the intestine and that they didn't cause toxicity, but new research is emerging that they have an impact on the system because they are converted back into their parent compound which has toxic effects[153] [154]. What protects the body is a healthy microbiome. However, these components in food damage the healthy bugs and make the body more susceptible to deleterious effects.

10. **The ferment in our foods.** Fermented foods are often touted as the end all and be all to improve your digestive D-Spot health. We take common foods and drinks, like cabbage, grains, grapes and green tea and ferment them. Fermented foods like alcohol including beers, liquors and wine, kimchi, kombucha, sauerkraut, yogurt and kefir are all the new health rage. Cheese, pickles and olives are also common foods that people don't realize are fermented. The issue with fermentation is that it can negatively affect the D-Spot indirectly. Fermentation releases histamine, a biogenic amine, that in certain cases has caused death[155]. Histamine is also an irritant, think if you rub against poison ivy, you get a major rash. That rash is caused by the

release of histamine. Histamine is directly linked to irritation, whether on the skin or the mucosal membrane of the D-Spot. Take as an example the FODMAP diet for irritable bowel syndrome. The FODMAP diet restricts all types of fermentable foods as well as certain foods that release histamine. Long term use of this diet can cause derangement of the microbiome[156]. We evolved with consuming fermented foods. The issue is that we are exposed in excess and other factors are also harming our D-Spot. This is why it's important to reintroduce these foods at the right time. In someone with a non-cooperative D-Spot, it's best to avoid these foods until the D-Spot has been healed and then re-introduce them so they can exert the goodness they were destined to provide.

11. **Your hormonal self.** Believe it or not, your hormones have a lot to do with the bugs you are harbouring in your D-Spot. We have maintained an evolutionary relationship with the bugs in our environment and that helps with the biological preservation of our systems through the orchestration of our hormones like estrogen, progesterone, and the glucocorticoids[157]. Candida albicans increase their ability to colonize with increasing levels of estradiol, one of the forms of estrogen in our bodies[158]. Many women using hormone replacement therapy or taking the birth control pill artificially increase the estrogen in their bodies and with that yeast overgrowth in both the vagina and the D-Spot. The dominating microbes on the mucous membrane of the vagina are determined by what we eat and what comes into our body. You wouldn't think those are connected but they are. The mucous membrane is the same across the entire system, from the oral, nasal, ear, vaginal, digestive, and anal canal. If you're having Candida yeast or other infections, that pattern is mimicked everywhere[159].

Pasteur invented the germ theory[160]. At the beginning of his career, the bug was everything. As things evolved, he realized that it was the system that made the difference. There is much controversy stating that on his death bed, Pasteur recanted his theory saying, "Claude Bernard, was right, 'the terrain is everything, the germ is nothing!'"[161]. Whether this is truth or simply speculation, we do not really know.

What we do know is that you create your gut environment by what you do, how you live, what you breathe and eat. The focus need not be on the bug, but how you can create a healthy vessel that only supports the healthy bugs.

Stressor 9: Quantity and Quality of your Food

The D-Spot is a delicate system. It seems that everywhere you look the health recommendation of five meals per day is the standard. Oh, and please make sure that you never ever skip breakfast. Those are the conventional thoughts of our time. The reality, in my opinion, is that it makes much more sense to listen to your body. Eat when you are hungry, less is better. Too much food, too many times during the day, and all you end up doing is stressing out your D-Spot.

I remember reading a wonderful book from my dear mentor, Deepak Chopra. His work has accompanied me throughout the thick and thin of my life. In naturopathic medical school, I would watch and rewatch his video on the <u>Seven Spiritual Laws of Success</u> as it just resonated strongly with my heart. It gave me hope through school, which was needed with all the dogma of an educational institution that can suck the living life out of you. Oh, Sh*t! I have always valued his opinion greatly because it just always makes sense. He follows the natural laws.

None of us were born yesterday. Our food, our nutrition, our nourishment, is an area of our lives that is so near and dear to our hearts. We know inherently what is good for us. As I was reading one of Deepak Chopra's books entitled <u>Overcoming Addiction</u>, something struck me. His knowledge and advice was just plain simple. Eat when you are hungry. Nice. I can do that. Shortly thereafter I stopped forcing myself to have breakfast because I realized it was futile. My body didn't want food upon waking, for that wasn't right for me. It may or may not be right for you. Evidence suggests that it doesn't matter when you consume your protein in a day, as long as you consume enough for your daily requirements for your system[162]. There is no specific time of the day to eat that is best, except when you are hungry. Teens are notorious for not being hungry in the morning and a systematic review of the research into the needs of children and adolescents, remains inconclusive with regards to demonstrating a cognitive benefit with breakfast[163]. The key point here is to listen to what your body wants.

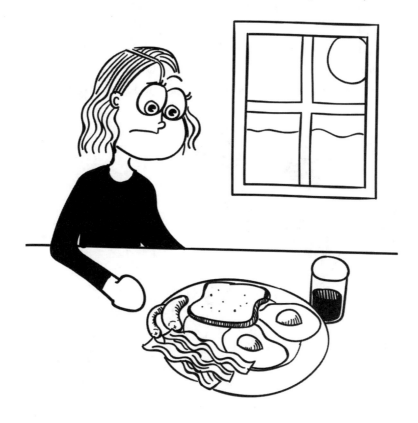

Hunger is an important signal of a physical need. Sometimes an emotional need can feel much like hunger. Geneen Roth explains this in detail in her book, Feeding the Hungry Heart. She discusses food used to cope with lack of emotional connection. Food is nourishment on many levels. It is emotional and nutritional. You can't force emotions and you can't force your eating. If you are eating according to other peoples' rules and not listening to your body, you push your digestion to work against your higher good.

Be a cougar, not a cow. Your D-Spot is a work horse, and because it works so hard, it deserves a break too. These days, you've been recommended by nutritionists and personal trainers to graze all day long. Grazing, however, is for cows and you don't want to look like a cow. You want to look like a cougar, lean and mean, feeding only after a good hunt. Eating all day long is for people that may be training all day long and are supremely physically active, as they need the constant input of calories. For most of us who are sedentary, we don't burn very many calories at all. We burn more calories fasting than we do eating, so we need to switch to more hours without food, and less of eating.

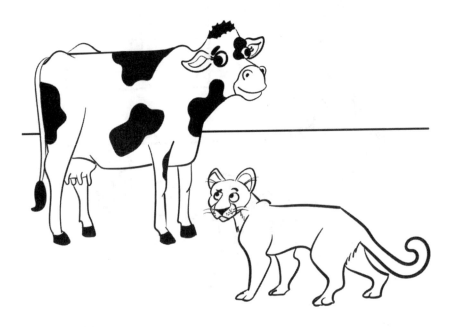

Don't eat a cookie while you vacuum. The principle behind this is simple. If you are constantly feeding, your body's energy is focused on digestion and not on its other jobs, such as the vitally important job of cleaning up and detoxifying. I look at it like this. Can you vacuum and eat a cookie at the same time? Absolutely not, because your cookie is going to crumble and make a mess of where you just vacuumed. You simply cannot do both at the same time. Although, according to some of my patients, they say it's the perfect scenario! Cleaning is such an important job in the body, because we are constantly (via biochemical reactions) making garbage and intaking garbage that all needs to come out. No time to take out the trash if you are feeding all day.

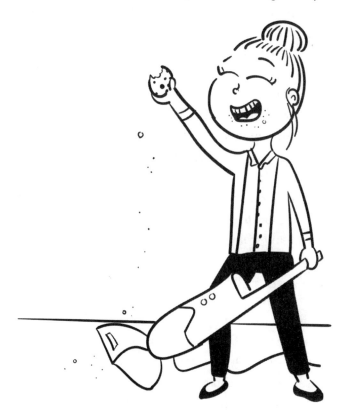

Food fits in your fist. The other major aspect of nourishment is that we eat too much. HARA HACHI BU is a Japanese dietetics principle that states to only eat until you are about 80% full. Amazing, if you consider our stomachs are the size of closed fists, how much in excess of what we should be having are we eating? Too much! Oh, Sh*t!

In this Super Size Me nation, our portion sizes are for large wildebeests and not the typical average female or male. We need to reassess our 'normals' in terms of sizes, as we are feeding too much and overloading our D-Spots. Start ordering one size lower than you did before. Over time, you will start to find that you fit into clothing that is one size lower than before.

Sit down. Take your time. Chew and enjoy your food. The highly popular Dukan Diet recommends something to its participants; take one hour to eat your food. Guess what happens to these people? Instead of gulping down their food in ten minutes, and then sitting there for fifty minutes waiting for the time to pass by, they learn to eat slowly. They chew and enjoy their food. When you do this, you get full faster and you are avoiding so many problems that come with gulping food down. When you gulp, you bloat like a goat, and overwhelm your D-Spot with highly undigested food. This is why I use my Grateful Dung™ Bracelet during meals. I put food into my mouth then I touch the Tiger's eye beads on the bracelet all the way around, with each bead representing one chew, until I make it back to where I started. Then I know that my food has been mechanically pre-digested enough to swallow, making my stomach's job easy!

Clearly quality. Food quality is of the utmost importance. You are feeding your temple of life. This is the one and only body that you have been given. There are no second chances. Feed it only the best. So many people gawk at the cost of organic, but it need not be just organic food that we are purchasing. Organic is obviously the ideal but there is a rule of thumb I use that I will explain later which will help you to work out whether you should buy local, imported, organic or conventional. The choice will be yours.

These factors impact your life in a major way, yet they are simply minor to implement. Take note of your practices and where you are at with the quantity and quality of your food and rate on a scale of 1-10.

Stressor 10: Supplements

When people take supplements, their intent is to improve the state of their health. Little do they know that sometimes these supplements are actually sinister and slimy, depleting their system. For activation they demand extra use of already low supplies of nutrients, their dosage is too low to have a therapeutic effect, or they don't break down properly, resulting in expensive urine and poop! Bluntly, many supplements don't do what they claim to do.

Having worked in the natural health industry for close to 20 years, you get to learn and see a thing or two about the quality of supplements. Like our food, supplements are not all created equally, and to most, without the discerning eye, you would simply go for the least expensive option. Buyer beware! You really do get what you pay for, especially when it comes to supplements. Be very critical of what you put into your system. I personally will only put the best in it, for both myself and my patients.

How do you know what is good and what is mediocre? A lot comes down to ingredients and how they are packaged.

Quality control. Supplement manufacturers need to stay on top of the highest standards for their nutrients and fillers. Reports have been made that certain supplements lack quality control standards, specifically as to the amount of the active components of the ingredients and the claims made on the label[164].

Fillers, food coloring and fermentation. Fillers are used to speed up the manufacturing process so pill filling machines don't get clogged, and in some cases, to actually enhance therapeutic effect. Which fillers are allowable? Many people have a gripe against magnesium stearate and I did too, until I began to do some research which actually changed my mind.

There is both a bovine source of magnesium stearate as well as a vegetable source. Magnesium stearate is naturally occurring in some of our foods like cocoa and flax seeds[165] [166]. As a stable compound that doesn't break down via digestion, there isn't a concern. But as with all things, it's what happens when you absorb it.

There is a potential for the magnesium portion of the magnesium stearate to actually exert a therapeutic effect. That's good news, since many of us are walking around with an undiagnosed magnesium deficiency[167]. The downside is that stearic acid is the predominant saturated fat in our diet and produced by our bodies. However, just because it's called a saturated fat, doesn't mean it's a bad guy. Stearic acid is not implicated in heart disease. In fact, it actually helps to lower your LDL, what we like to call your lousy cholesterol[168].

One thing's for sure, the dose that you get of magnesium stearate is very low in most supplements, somewhere between 0.25-1.5% of total capsule weight, that correlates to about 5 mg in a 500mg tablet[169].

Ideally, your supplements have absolutely no fillers, but this is only possible if they are compounded by hand. Something is needed to keep things moving smoothly, so why not fat? Other options that are used are silica, L-leucine, and microcrystalline cellulose which all seem to have low impact as well.

What is not necessary, is to use a multitude of fillers as well as food coloring agents. A very popular children's vitamin, which I'm sure we have all taken at one point in time and dates back to a prehistoric cartoon, has 39 non-medicinal filler ingredients along with food coloring. Oh, Sh*t! A popular adult vitamin contains 18 non-medicinal fillers and food colorings. I like to ask myself at this point, "How is there enough room for the vitamins and minerals, if it's a one-a-day dosage?"

Time to start looking at labels and learning key ingredients. One easy rule is that if you can't pronounce it, might not be a good idea to ingest it.

Activated nutrients. Many times the ingredients used are the cheapest form of the nutrient. The company hasn't stayed up to date on the research, in terms of what is the best nutrient for optimal interaction in the body. Or they just want to save money and improve their bottom line to the detriment of your health.

We want the vitamin or nutrient to already be activated before ingested. Otherwise, a non-activated nutrient will deplete your vitamin resources because you have to use up vital nutrients and minerals to make it active. This is basically working against yourself. We need to hold the companies that we purchase our health supplements from up to the highest standards that only allow them to produce the best of the best. An example of this is vitamin B12. This is a quick way to check if your supplements are royalty or rascals under cover. There are three forms of B12. Listed from most expensive to least expensive; methylcobalamin, hydroxycobalamin and cyanocobalamin. Pick up and read the ingredients on the supplements you are currently taking. Nine times out of ten you will find your supplements contain the cheapest form cyanocobalamin, unless you are a highly enlightened health seeker and already knew this, then your supplements would contain methylcobalamin, the highest quality, quickly absorbed and already active form of B12. It'll go right into your body and start doing its job immediately.

Cyanocobalamin on the other hand, the cheap, most common form put into low quality supplements needs to be converted by the body in order to do its job. The cobalamin, which is the B12, is complexed with cyano, which is cyanide, so your body needs to cleave that component out and then detoxify the cyanide. This process requires using valuable vitamins from your body to get it out of the system. Seems like a waste of time and too much work for nothing!

Therapeutic dosage. Many times the formulas contain so little of each of the ingredients that they exert no effect. You may as well be drinking water. You will notice many formulas on the store shelves with a multitude of ingredients. All of the ingredients are typically used in dealing with a certain condition, so the formula just sounds superb! In naturopathic medicine, however, we have a tendency to avoid combination formulas, unless they are very well made, because we usually dose the nutrient on its own. To exert a physiological effect, you need a very specific dose. I look at it like this. If you are a 130-170 lb person, do you think a tiny fairy dust sampling of so and so herb, is going to do anything in your system? I think not! To exert a big change you require a large enough amount. At this point in the research, we have a clearer idea as to the therapeutic dosages. Take the catechins in green tea, EGCG. Approximately 600-900 mg is required per day to help with the reduction of metabolic syndrome in adults[170]. In many combination formulas you're lucky if you get 100mg. You would have to take six to nine capsules in order to get a therapeutic dosage! In general, many combination formulas sound good in theory, but unless you are taking enough of them and know what the therapeutic benchmark is, they can just be a waste of money.

Breakdown-ability. Many times the formulas are placed into non-absorbable forms, like tablets. Tablets are referred to by Dr. Julian Whitaker in the The Great Vitamin Hoax as "Bed Pan Bullets". Nurses see a few two many of these in bed pans of hospitals. These forms of compressed tablets are difficult to digest and people tend to eliminate them out with little to no absorption.

This is a major issue, as sometimes people are spending hundreds of dollars on their supplements and not getting what they are expecting out of them. Worse still, if they are trying to treat a chronic progressive disease where they need to see action rapidly.

I am a self proclaimed supplement 'Sh*t Disturber'. Nothing gets into my clinic, my mouth or down my patients throats, unless I would personally take it. I've done my time taking low grade supplements and I won't do it again. You think you are saving money, but you are just wasting both time and money and getting no effect. Sometimes these supplements can actually deplete you of your own nutrient stores!

Choose your supplements wisely. They are not all made the same and remember, you get what you pay for. Rate your supplements stress at the end of this chapter.

Stressor 11: Environmental Toxins

Industrialization dramatically increased the disturbance on our D-Spots. Some chemicals have become highly popularized like Bisphenol A (BPA), a plastic used in manufacturing. It has been categorized as an environmental obesogen because of many of its impacts on our bodies, one being the shifting of the gut microbiome[171]. This isolated chemical is only one of the 130 million plus chemicals that have been added to the CAS registry to date.

We are exposed each and every second of our lives to contaminants and we don't even know the full effect they have on our bodies. It's hard to avoid and difficult to even list everything to which we are exposed. From plasticizers in your shower curtain, industrial solvents/lubricants that make your memory foam mattress, additives in food to preserve its freshness, agricultural chemicals that keep the bugs out of our crops and feeds, pharmaceutical agents like birth control pills and antidepressants that pollute our water supply. These hopefully enlighten you to a few.

Even things that we drink, eat and put on our bodies that we assume are healthy can be contaminated. Our healthy foods that we eat, like teas, depending on which source they come from, can be more toxic than expected.

In Japan, tea leaves are allowed to have 50 ppm of neonicotinoids, the pesticide responsible for killing the bees of the world. This level is much higher than in other parts of the world[172]. With tea being such an important export and something that we consume from this part of the world, you may reconsider having that next cup of matcha ceremonial green tea from Japan, its one of the reasons I don't prescribe it.

Rice and fish are food products that are recognized to be contaminated with higher levels of metals such as cadmium, arsenic, mercury, lead and cobalt. A study of a population on a gluten free diet, who tend to eat more rice and fish, revealed that these people actually had higher levels of the metals than their counterparts eating a diet containing gluten[173]. This is concerning as many people are jumping on the bandwagon and following a gluten free diet for their health, but it may not actually be the healthiest if you are substituting rice!

Clothing made from organic cotton is still sprayed with polybrominated flame retardants that are toxic to our health. So, although we may be benefitting from the lack of pesticides on the organic clothing, we are still getting exposure to chemicals. These polybrominated flame retardants are notorious for being absorbed through the skin[174], ultimately adding to the stress on our system.

Your rayon clothing accumulates 3-10x more volatile compounds that are within the air such as phthalates that are added to perfumes, and halogenated flame retardants! So plastic clothing really is worse for you[175].

Another study looked at how clothing transfers phthalate esters, brominated flame retardants (BFRs) and organophosphate esters (OPEs)[176] and how clothing is an efficient transporter of these chemicals into laundry water. So wearing clothing makes us part of the vehicle for transfer of chemicals.

Dietary and treatment oils like olive oil and castor oil are often packaged in plastic and absorb chemicals from the bottles they are stored in. Castor oil is by far the worst affected by plastic because it is a carrier oil. Never purchase your oils in plastic, especially the queen of oils, castor oil.

You simply can't run and you can't hide! The negative effect of a chemical introduced by our diet[177] affects our D-Spot by altering our genes, or has effects that are even more far-reaching that may alter metabolism and induce diabetes[178]. The jury is clear, these environmental contaminants have far more reaching effects than what we even know at this point, including a negative effect on our D-Spots.

Add up the total of stressors on your system.

Rate your Sugar STRESS:

Low Stress   High Stress

1 2 3 4 5 6 7 8 9 10

Rate your Alcohol STRESS:

Low Stress   High Stress

1 2 3 4 5 6 7 8 9 10

Rate your Processed Food STRESS:

Low Stress   High Stress

1 2 3 4 5 6 7 8 9 10

Rate your Caffeine STRESS:

Low Stress   High Stress

1 2 3 4 5 6 7 8 9 10

Rate your Starvation STRESS:

Low Stress   High Stress

1 2 3 4 5 6 7 8 9 10

Rate your Food Sensitivity STRESS:

Low Stress   High Stress

1 2 3 4 5 6 7 8 9 10

Rate your Emotional STRESS:

Low Stress   High Stress

1 2 3 4 5 6 7 8 9 10

Rate your Dysbiotic D-Spot:

Low Stress   High Stress

1 2 3 4 5 6 7 8 9 10

Rate your Q&Q of Food in your D-Spot:

Low Stress   High Stress

1 2 3 4 5 6 7 8 9 10

Rate your Supplements STRESS:

Low Stress   High Stress

1 2 3 4 5 6 7 8 9 10

Rate your Environmental STRESS:

Low Stress   High Stress

1 2 3 4 5 6 7 8 9 10

In this chapter you got an intimate look at the dynamics of the D-Spot and how the body can easily be affected by multiple factors. You have complete control over many and also a choice to avoid them. Some, you do not. Now that we know what can affect you, let's see how your D-Spot is responding.

CHAPTER 5

YOUR D-SPOT - DIVINE, DREARY OR DERANGED?

Life should be dynamic, and so should your D-Spot. Dynamic means happy. There is an ebb and flow of functions. Typically, that is breaking down and absorbing, packaging the waste and voiding.

Assessing the health of your D-Spot means looking deeper than just the symptoms that you are presently experiencing. It's about your entire life and body, day to day, not just what is physically happening in your D-Spot. There are many symptoms outside of the D-Spot that tell you whether it's dynamic or disturbed.

Stools are the first gateway to intimately knowing your D-Spot. To set our example as to what a good stool is, I encourage all of my patients to look at nature. If you have a dog, they are the best example. They eat and then poop, one to three times per day, depending on the feeding patterns of the dog. Fortunately for dogs, all they have to do is eat, sleep, poop, love and be loved back. Pretty much, it's the most zen life one could ask for, making it easy for the D-Spot to be divine.

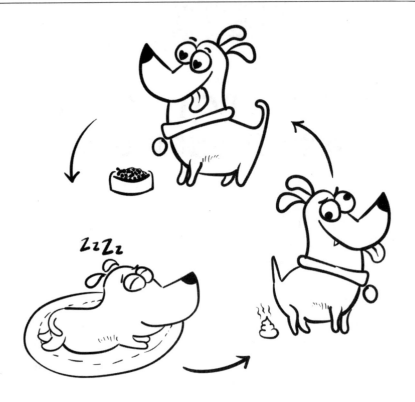

Because you may not live the life of a dog, you must become your own best **Poolice**! Your mission is to serve and protect your body and completely understand what is going on down there (pun completely intended). A sort of detective work is required to keep the peace.

Let's face it. A constipated person is a cranky person, unhappy and miserable. Someone who has proper flow feels good and is happy with life. Someone who can't keep it together isn't happy either. He may know where every single toilet is because he can't stay solid. That's no way to live. So let's learn what's normal, what's not, and why.

I could be conventional and use the medically recommended Bristol Stool Chart for analyzing stools, but I like to do things differently. That's one of the reasons I'm a naturopath! In my practice, I've decided to simplify and make it fun in order for it to be memorable and to help you really grasp the concepts and laugh too, which, by the way, is also medicine!

So to start, what is considered a normal stool, or what I like to call a Royal Flush? These are the terms used to describe normal stools.

Timing and Frequency: Pooping should be a daily practice. It's similar to the dog, timed after you eat. Alternatively, first thing in the morning because that is when you are the most relaxed. Anywhere between one to three times per day is optimal. Food comes in and should be moving things out.

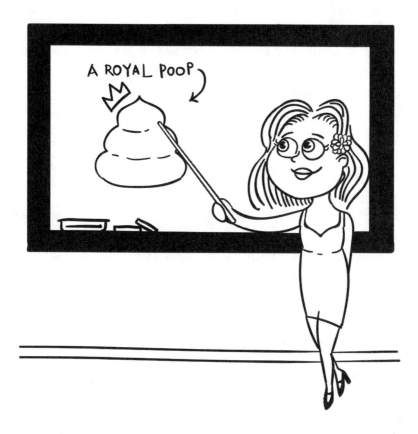

Size: The ideal stool size is roughly 12 inches long, from your wrist to your elbow. If you place your left elbow at your ribcage and bring your arm down into the centre of your belly, that's the length of the descending colon, and likely the food you ate 24 hrs ago. That would be the ideal daily elimination. It can be produced all at once or at different times throughout the day. You could have three 4 inch stools, two 6 inch stools or one 12 incher. You get to be the artist on this one.

Consistency: The stool should be solid and come out in one healthy strand, which looks just like a ginormous king size sausage, no cow plops, pebbles, strands that are flat or thin, or liquid-like loungers are allowed.

Color: Stools should be any shade of brown. Light brown, dark brown, medium brown... these are all normal. If your stool is anything outside of this shade, it is cause for concern. Green stools are an indication of low stomach acid or infection by virus or bacteria. White, red or black stools are medical emergencies and if you see them in your throne you should seek medical attention immediately. An awesome tool to use as a guide is the Queen of the Thrones™ Grateful Dung™ Bracelet. It is made with Tigers eye stone beads that reflect the spectrum of browns that are healthy colors of stool. You can find the Grateful Dung™ Bracelet on my website, www.drmarisol.com.

Feel: Here, I don't mean for you to touch it, but if you're feeling adventurous, go for it! Just make sure to wash up afterwards. Feeling is how it squeezes out of your body. It's ideal to feel it coming out smoothly, like butter, with no straining or turtle necking. Turtle necking is usually described as your stool peeping out and then going back in. It should all come out with one gentle squeeze, like toothpaste coming out of the tube. You should feel as though you can't believe what came out of you once you take a peek!

Wiping: Wiping once with nothing on the toilet paper seems abnormal but really it isn't. If you think about it, indigenous cultures had no toilet paper. They simply walk through the hot dry land, squat and then pop! The only thing left for them to clean their bums with is dry brush, not exactly soft on their cheeks. But the fact is, they don't really need it, because there is no wiping necessary. There would be nothing on the paper. Plop an indigenous person into the Standard North American (SAD) diet and they are sure to become a "Hyper Wiper" in no time.

In the bowl and bathroom: Your precious discharge should leave no evidence. It should sink to the bottom of the throne, leaving no skid marks. The smell should be sucked away on flushing. If not, you know that your pipes need a good cleaning.

In total there are 11 criteria or as I like to call them 'Golden Nuggets' that can be used to analyze your stools for signs of nutrient deficiencies, hormone imbalances, nervous system issues and digestive problems. They can be found on www.drmarisol.com in my e-book, Know Your Poo.

To get a free download of one of the Golden Nuggets, the 50 Shades of Poo, check out the resource page at the back of the book.

The best tool to remind you to peek after you poo is my one and only After you Poo Parfum™, **Eau de Throne**™. It is an organic spray created with top quality essential oils of lavender, rosemary, clove and citrus. Conventional air fresheners and plug-ins contain toxins that are harmful to the D-Spot, so I wanted to design a spray that is totally safe and effective. It smells absolutely amazing and the essential oils help to calm and relax the body, so you can have legendary bowel movements, plus they cleanse the air so that you don't leave your bacteria hanging around for the next person! You can leave the throne with an odor you are sure to own. Visit www.drmarisol.com to get yours today!

So now that you've read, heard and laughed a little about what comes out of you, let's kick it up a notch. I want you to never forget and to understand what it all means. To know what is good and what is not-so-hot, nothing paints the picture better than a picture. I want you to look into the bowl each and every time you go and know exactly what is going on down under.

Get to know the Legends of the Throne!

(Check out the resource page at the back of this book for a link to download in color)

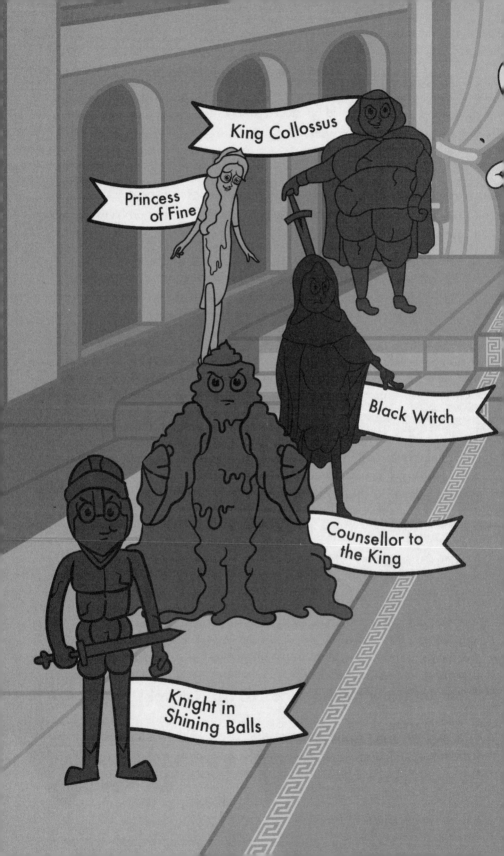

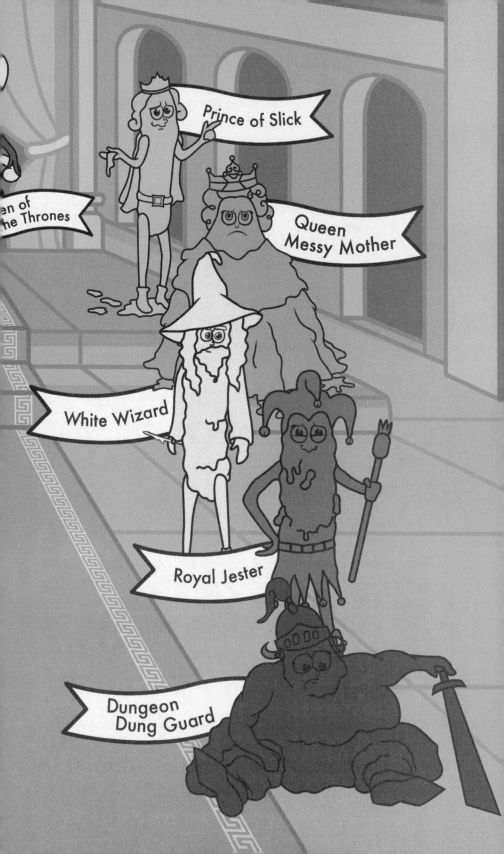

1. Queen of the Thrones

The queen is a beautiful sight to behold and a pleasure to meet! Most call her perfect as she slides out like butter into the throne. She's perfectly curvy and never leaves a skid mark or bad stench behind. When you wipe it is oh-so-clean and she sinks down into the depths without a trace. She is firm and thick, and measures the length of your elbow to your wrist. If you're healthy, then she's making an appearance daily, owning your throne and helping you to feel lighter and brighter!

2. Knight in Shining Balls

Made of balls of steel, he fights to protect the throne. All of his fighting is a sign of stress in your body and depleted levels of magnesium. It's also an indication that you haven't been drinking enough water.

3. Royal Jester

He peeks out, always with a surprise on the outside. Sometimes unrecognizable debris, sometimes a perfectly intact piece of food, the jester likes to keep you guessing. His appearance is a sign of maldigestion and low digestive enzymes.

4. King Collossus

King Collossus is compacted, enormous and difficult to pass. He shows up for those who over indulge in meat and wine but forget about fiber and water. He visits the throne from time to time but takes so long to get there. He makes you feel as if you are birthing a poo baby! NOT very comfortable.

5. Princess of Fine

This princess is so fine and delicate she's always afraid to be seen. When she shows up, thin as a rack, it's a sign that you're stressed to the max. She follows a very thin line but when the pressure hits she falls apart on impact. She's a sign of digestion problems like inflammation, mucus and food sensitivities - like she just can't relax under the pressure of being a princess.

6. Prince of Slick

The prince is so slimy and always gloating and floating. He leaves an oil slick trail in his path as he tries to claim the throne and causes you to hyper wipe. He is a sign of not digesting your fats properly, issues with your gall bladder or lack of digestive enzymes.

7. The Queen Messy Mother

Once legendary, and now losing it, she always comes out a wet mess. She splatters onto the throne, reminiscent of the day she once owned it. She has many issues and indicates stress and a transit time that is much too fast.

8. Dungeon Dung Guard

This dungeon dweller hasn't seen the light of day. Sitting in the dungeon, he looks like a plop of cow dung and is sad and depressed. The dungeon is so damp and moist, an environment where bad bugs like yeast and Candida run rampant. Inflammation, food allergies and sensitivities are common when you see this guy, and hyper wiping is usually a given.

9. Counsellor to the King

He's the most sinister in the kingdom, but hides it so well. He sticks to the throne cause he's so full of mucus, but behind the scenes it's all bad news. He's red like the devil, and always out for blood (a sign of bleeding in the lower digestive tract). **Seek medical attention** before this conniving scoundrel does you in.

10. Black Witch

All dressed in black, she comes out as a bearer of bad news. When she's around she seems to bring out the worst in people, so if you see her, **run to your doctor immediately**. She is a sign of bleeding in the upper digestive tract and you need get checked out!

11. White Wizard

The white wizard, magical and whimsical, is actually a very ominous sign. It typically indicates a blockage in the upper abdomen, not allowing bile to dump into the intestines and color stools. He is a **medical emergency** - do not take it lightly, his magical spells are a major cause for concern! Always seek medical attention if prolonged, uncomfortable or if you are unsure. Your doctor is your health partner, involve them!

Other Telltale Signs from your D-Spot…

Facts from the Farts

Another way of knowing how balanced your D-Spot is, is by how your farts smell and the type of gas that you are producing. Depending on the critters living in your D-Spot, they are a dead giveaway of what's gone wrong. These are hypotheses based on personal and professional experience as well as naturopathic practice and reported from the teachings of Dr. Dickson Thom.

You can hear it but you can't smell it - The loud ones come on with a bang but leave little lingering behind. The lack of smell is simply that this toot is made up of hydrogen gas. They come from the first part of the colon known as the ascending colon on the right side of your body. It runs from your right hip up to your right ribcage. These gas leaks are also typically correlated to carbohydrate maldigestion.

Smelly Nellies and Lingering Lovelies - These toots tell a tale of protein maldigestion and likely low stomach acid. As the food moves down the D-Spot, the bacterial profile changes. The difference in the smell just depends on what part of the colon is having the problem.

- If you have a major methane smelling fart, A.K.A. "smelly nellies", that remind you of driving in the country after the cow manure has been laid on the fields. These are coming from your transverse colon that reaches from the bottom of the right ribcage to the bottom of the left ribcage.

- When your gas is silent but deadly, then you are having hydrogen sulphide farts. They could be compared to rotten eggs.

What About the Bloat?

Bloating is a sensitive issue for those that experience it. If you deal with it in your D-Spot, you are not a happy camper as it can be very uncomfortable. Some people bloat so much that they look as though they are pregnant. This can happen to females and males of all ages.

If you are only bloated after food and wake with a flat stomach, this can be caused by low or a lack of digestive enzymes for a certain type of food, i.e. fat, carbohydrates or protein, or a combination of those foods. Your stomach is flat in the morning because your body has had enough time to "clean out the food".

If you are bloated constantly, even on waking, then your issues are based on a severe problem with gut bacteria. Your D-Spot has been overrun by bad bugs causing major inflammation and irritation. Your work needs to focus on changing your entire gut microbiome (the environment in your gut). This is classically referred to as small intestine bacterial overgrowth, or SIBO for short.

Bloating, depending on how long after eating, will signal different areas of your body that are affected.

1. **Right after meals signals** issues with your digestion and specifically the stomach with low stomach acid and digestive enzymes.

2. **Bloating one hour after eating** typically signals bad bug overgrowth in the small and large intestine.

The body is an incredible system that will tell you all you need to know. But, only if you are open to receiving the messages.

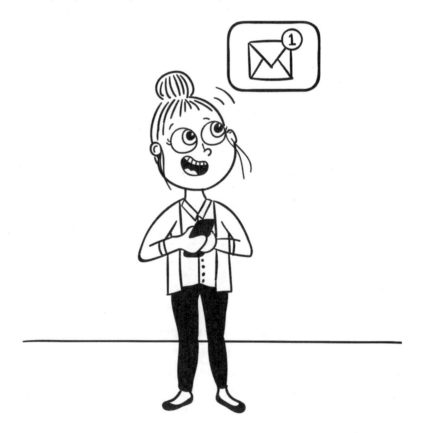

Principles - Natural Laws

Natural systems all have warning mechanisms. They present themselves as decay or failures in the synchronicity of working parts. They lose their ability to work as smoothly as they once did. The signs are plenty, and your body has many ringtones, notifications and signals that you need to become aware of, so you can be an informed owner of your only temple. This is why when assessing your D-Spot health, you can't ignore symptoms and signs from other "parts" of your body. Why? Because you are a whole ecosystem.

Grade your D-Spot Health - Is your D-Spot Dynamic, Dull or Dreary?

This questionnaire takes into account all of the measures that we have just discussed including bowel movements, bloating and gas production. Fill this questionnaire out with honesty, because that will help you the most.

There are four areas to measure and grade your D-Spot. The A's, B's, C's and D's of the D-Spot.

A = Appetite - It is healthy and balanced. You eat and are full. You are completely satisfied with your meal.

B = Behaviour - You are balanced in both body and mind. You eat your food and slowly enjoy each delicious mouthful. Never too fast, yet not excessively slow.

C = Clearing - Elimination is at its best and you more often see the Queen of the Thrones™ rather than the Prince of Slick or the Royal Jester.

D = Digestion - Your digestion is easy and breezy. You consume and it makes no impact on your body except that of feeling fabulous and energized, with no bloating and no gas.

A and **B** category questions are based on the gut-mind connection, ie. how well your nervous system communicates with your D-Spot. People whose score is heavily weighted in this regard have a **nervous gut**. So their problem is more mental, so to say. Their communication from their brains to their D-Spots isn't smooth. In fact, it is often compromised by things that have nothing to do with digestion, such as love life drama!

C and **D** category questions are based more on physiology, so there is likely a problem with the bacteria and mechanism of the gut. With these category questions there actually is an issue with the functioning of the gut.

Depending on which category you are more concentrated on will be your dominant type. The overall score will be your indicator of the degree of dysfunction in your D-Spot, and will be a guide to how many times a year you should repeat this six week program.

e D-Spot Quiz

ve yourself a score to each of
e following statements.

ts..never
ts..sometimes
ts..always

petite is Just Right
questions)   /10

Never feel full
Hungry all the time — eat like a horse
Never feel hungry — eat like a bird
Intense cravings
Have a negative association with food — judge
all your food as bad or good

havior at its Best
7 Questions)

Scarf down your food
Don't chew your food
Craving for chocolate (possible magnesium
deficiency)
Craving for sugars, pop, candy and junk food
(yeast imbalance, bad gut bugs)
Craving pastries, cookies, breads and pastas
(possible serotonin deficiency)
Craving for protein (possible lack of
neurotransmitters, sugar/insulin unbalanced)
Craving for caffeine in coffee, soda, black tea
or energy drinks (possible dopamine
deficiency)
Craving for salt (adrenals)
Craving for wheat and dairy (opiate
addiction)
Cravings for fats (possible hormone or fat
deficiency)
Eat more when stressed
Eat less when stressed
Tired after meals
Can't let go of problems easily
Binging
Purging
Have anxiety, depression or mental health
disorder

/34

Clearance of Crap (21 questions)
__ Frequent diarrhea (more than 3x/day, and
more than 3x/week)
__ Frequent constipation (less than 6 bowel
movements/week)
__ Alternating constipation and diarrhea
__ Turtle-necking stools (comes out and goes back
in)
__ Incomplete evacuation (never feel empty)
__ Mucous
__ Blood
__ Undigested food
__ Cow plops
__ Skid marks in bowl
__ Oil in water of toilet bowl
__ Floating stools
__ Repetitively thin stools
__ Rabbit pellets
__ Large, hard stool that is painful to pass
__ Green
__ Grey/white
__ Black
__ Red (not associated with beets)
__ Hyper wiping
__ Itchy bum   /42

Digestion — Symptoms of D-Spot Drama (21 questions)
__ Blue-eyed
__ Ringing in the ears/tinnitus
__ Foggy brain
__ Itchy ears
__ Post-nasal drip
__ Sinus congestion
__ Bad breath
__ Burping
__ Reflux/GERD
__ Bloating
__ Gas
__ Bellyaches
__ Vaginal discharge or infection
__ Urinary tract infections
__ Skin rashes, plaques or generally irritated skin
__ Waking at night to urinate
__ Increased frequency of urination
__ Green tea makes you nauseous on an empty
stomach
__ Supplements on an empty stomach make you
nauseous
__ Red cheeks or rosacea
__ Nose swollen (Rhinophyma)   /42

ld:
pts — if you have a hormonal diagnosis, such as menopause, PMS, endometriosis, or a thyroid condition_____
pts — if you have an immune diagnosis, such as Hashimoto's Thyroiditis, cancer, rheumatoid arthritis _____
al of 64 questions plus the hormonal or immune component.

al A: _____ Total B: _____ Total C: _____ Total D: _____

al A + B + C + D + extras = _____ (max of 148 points)

ur D-Spot Score:

0 = Divine D-Spot   40-90 = Dreary D-Spot   90+ = Deranged D-Spot

Why is there not a specific type, or category into which I fall? It's simply because the human body is distinct and unique in every person. Categorizing only leads to issues. Each of us is on a very individualized spectrum of D-Spot health.

So, based on your score, is your D-Spot **divine, dreary** or **deranged**?

Please note that some answers may be considered medical emergencies. If you're unsure or your condition has been going on for a long time without having proper medical follow-up, please make an appointment with your health care provider immediately in order to figure things out.

Go to www.drmarisol.com/d-spot-quiz/ for an online version of this questionnaire.

So now that you have your number and you've found out where you are on the D-Spot divine to deranged spectrum, you know how many times per year you want to repeat this three step program.

Divine = Once a year (ideally in the spring)
Dreary = Twice a year (ideally in the spring and fall)
Deranged = Four times a year (every season)

D-Spot from Deranged to Divine

There are three steps to take in order to get your D-Spot feeling its best. The first time you do this plan, you will spend two weeks focusing on each step. As you repeat the program, step one and step three will become second nature to you, and you'll only need to repeat step two of the program (Clean like a Queen) once, twice, or four times a year, depending on your D-Spot score.

Step One: Connect like a Cavewoman

The focus here is on getting in tune with your natural rhythms, getting back to your ancestral paleolithic ways, getting your bowels moving, starting a supplement regime and beginning the clean up that drives all healing. This step should take two weeks.

Step Two: Clean like a Queen

What you should be eating to heal your gut, the food combinations that heal instead of harm, and then supplements to help treat the gut. The Clean phase is where we delve into the D-Spot Meal Practice, and lasts two weeks. For best results (and when you repeat this program next time) extend this phase to 4-6 weeks.

Step Three: Calm like Buddha

Learn the keys to keeping it together in the longterm and how to listen to your body to understand which foods bug you upon reintroduction. How to keep your gut cells kissing; let go of leaky gut promoting practices and adopt new health practices of stress management, a regular supplement regime, castor oil packs and a balance between indulgence and discipline. Take two weeks to master this phase and adopt it into your everyday life.

Health Practices To Last A Lifetime

The reason for the stages is to develop a mind-blowing D-Spot and have it all of the time. In general, it can take three weeks to three months to develop and maintain a habit. In fact, research also shows that for a habit to be adopted more rapidly, having the hormone cortisol in your system is beneficial. Research has shown that in the morning when your cortisol is naturally the highest, you learn a habit 50 days faster than in the evening. It'll take 105.95 days in the morning to solidify it as opposed to 154.01 in the evening when your cortisol is lowest[179]. Why do I bring this up here? Simply because the process of changing can be stressful and can increase your stress hormone levels. But guess what? That is nature's magic at its finest. That will help you with your goals.

Think of it like this. To mold metal, you must stress it with fire. This creates a quick change because there is an enormous amount of stress. Water, on the other hand, changes things over time by consistent action, consistent friction and small consistent doses of a wee bit of stress.

So, if you want to mold yourself into the very best version of you, you need to add either an enormous amount of stress or be consistent and repetitive; like fire or like water. You need to focus on building lifestyle practices that will keep your D-Spot divine. I want you to be able to finish this program and in six weeks, feel a very different 'you'.

It will take a total of six weeks for the program the first time around, then a few final months to seal the deal, and you will feel the difference. As you transition back into normal life, you will find you feel like a very different you. With different taste buds, improved digestion and the ability to implement the Discipline Indulgence Principle in all areas of your life.

This is not meant to treat, cure or prevent any disease. Before undertaking any new health strategies ask your higher power, your gut, and your doctor if it is right for you. These are the protocols that I have used successfully with patients and are meant for education purposes only.

Ready? Let's get dirty... Time to dig in!

CHAPTER 6

CONNECT LIKE A CAVEWOMAN

Step one in healing your D-Spot is all about returning to the principle of connecting to your body and its natural rhythms which will greatly help you find optimal balance in your D-Spot. It's all about getting back to your cavewoman roots! Back to your original way! There you go, that's all folks...

This phase should last approximately two weeks. This is the minimum amount of time required to create a habit. Each portion of this book is written so that you can do different stages every two weeks. This way, the habits will build on each other, and it'll make it super easy to implement into your present lifestyle. At the end of six weeks, the goal is for you to have collected a number of very valuable tools that will serve you for life. They will help you to manage your health long-term.

Remember, with great effort you will achieve great change. So it just depends on how ready you are to live a different life. You can do this. We can do this together.

Following the same principles as you would to build your house and orchestrate a home, we will work through the Connect phase. For the D-Spot to heal, we must create the environment for it to be in a good space. That environment needs to be moving properly, ie. the energy flow has to be good. The D-Spot also has to be calm, and it has to be in tune, which means there needs to be an ebb and flow of the harmonies and melodies of life. The circadian rhythm regulation is of the utmost importance during this phase. Feeling energy when you wake and having a restful night's sleep is of the utmost importance.

People don't realize that sleep isn't simply just a commodity, it is such a necessity. During sleep, we can clean and heal, and therefore these are the foundations of the first step.

Our goals for the Connect phase are simple:

1. Get to know your D-Spot

2. Move what your mother gave you

3. Reset your day-night cycles

During your first two weeks, the focus will be on getting the timing of your life right.

Fasting Practice - Fast to Feast, Fast Till You Feast

Before you can do anything, first reduce the amount of garbage coming into your home. Most food is not considered garbage. However, when you are constantly eating and foraging, not abiding by the natural laws of having a set schedule and rhythm, you simply tend to eat more.

We have evolved that way, it's in our DNA which was programmed thousands of years ago, because we were not sure when our next meal would come. So your very first step is to reduce the amount of times that you eat and set yourself up on a schedule, so that you can entrain your body to an optimal feeding pattern. How this is done is by including periods of therapeutic fasting throughout your day.

Fasting helps to clean things up. I like to think of it like this. **Don't eat a cookie while you are vacuuming**, because the crumbs will get all over the place and you will simply have to keep on vacuuming. Taking a food break lets your body cleanse. Cleansing is the first step to helping things move in the right direction.

To keep things simple and easy for people, I propose to all my patients, "Just skip breakfast!" Yes, that's right, I want you to skip the "most important" meal of the day. Most of my patients have to pick themselves off the ground from the initial shock of my being a doctor and actually telling them to go against everything they have ever heard about nutrition. Many patients already aren't eating breakfast, they feel guilty telling me that they skip it all the time and they simply don't know what to think. I do, however, often see them breathe a sigh of relief when I tell them that they aren't hurting themselves by skipping breakfast. In fact, I've just freed them from this common misconception to understand that they may actually be helping themselves!

Let me explain how this works. It's really simple. Our bodies clean when we are not eating. Fasting is one of the longest observed health practices, much like taking a shower and washing or a baptism. Fasting is present in most cultures, think of lent and ramadan. I like to think of fasting as how we help to wash our insides by giving them a "food break".

The easiest way to add a fast into your health practice is to simply extend the amount of time that you actually "break the fast". Instead of eating within the first hour of waking, we recommend for you to see if you can extend the time up to 16 hours from the last meal you had the night before. In essence, you are still having breakfast, however you are just extending the time at which you have it.

The reason some of my patients, and perhaps you, are not having breakfast is because your body needs to clean, so therefore you are not hungry first thing in the morning. I tell my patients they are doing exactly what their bodies want and need, and good for them for listening! More time away from food means more efficient internal cleaning.

For some people, the morning fast simply does not work. Those with severe burn out or adrenal weakness and certain hormonal problems can find themselves more debilitated with fasting in the a.m. You can only find out by experimenting, or consulting your naturopathic doctor who may run urinary, saliva or blood tests for your adrenals and hormones.

See the resource page at the back of this book for a link to a lab that I use and trust. For these people, we simply switch the time of the fast. Some people will stop eating by 3 or 4 pm and will fast before bed and throughout their sleep, then feed in the a.m. Either way works, you just need to find the timing that works for you.

After you have fasted for about eight hours without food, your body turns on super cleaning mode. That's where your body will break down toxins, move them out and start to switch your metabolism to fat burning mode, which further eliminates the toxins that are stored in fat. So you not only get the benefit of breaking down fat, but you also benefit from reducing and removing toxins that are stored in your body.

Fat is the major storage zone for toxicity, so I never recommend more than 16 hours, because longer fasts can break down too much fat and release too many toxins that you may not be able to process and eliminate at this point in your D-Spot program.

One awesome benefit of fasting is that it seems to have the ability to improve your memory and reduce neurological inflammation[180]. This is probably one of the reasons that fasting has become so hip these days. With an ever increasing aging population, dementia, Alzheimer's and all types of neurological conditions are common and difficult to treat. Small lifestyle changes, like fasting, can be a major help.

An important part during the morning fast, is to make sure you are hydrating with plenty of **green tea,** herbal teas and water! Sorry, not COFFEE!!!! There are certain do's and drops for the fasting period. Here are the do's and drops to help you achieve your goals.

I know this can be tough to do, especially as many of us have learned to "eat like a king in the morning, lunch like a prince and dinner like a pauper". We are here to flip that philosophy on its head and your health.

Your most important 'do' during your FAST!

Fasting Do #1: Drown the D-Spot with Green Tea - Drop the Coffee and Other Sources of Caffeine

Caffeine in beverages such as coffee, soft drinks and energy drinks are a major culprit to drama in the D-Spot. Caffeine is detrimental to your nervous system balance and stresses out your system in the short term, causing hyperglycemia[181], a state of high blood sugar in your body. It irritates your gut lining and in the long term increases weight gain in the belly, causing many metabolic disturbances.

Caffeinated beverages are not all created equal. Coffee, as an example, does have certain aspects that are health promoting. It is known to improve mental clarity and in some studies can reduce the risk of diabetes via elements such as chlorogenic acid[182]. This is a phenolic compound, that lowers blood glucose concentrations[183] because it reduces absorption of glucose from the mucosa of the intestine by filling up the receptors, and not allowing glucose to transport from the D-Spot into the blood. The two important enzymes in the brush border membrane vesicles that get blocked are the glucose-6-phosphate translocase and the sodium-dependent glucose transport[184]. Although reducing blood sugar levels is good in terms of reducing risk of diabetes, this leaves the sugar to wreak havoc in the D-Spot by disturbing the ecology and feeding the bad bugs such as yeast and other invaders.

Furthermore, there is still much controversy as to the exact mechanism of reducing blood sugar as mentioned above. Another strong meta-analysis showed that in healthy male subjects, acute intake of caffeine from coffee increased hyperglycaemia and reduced insulin sensitivity[185]. Either way, it seems coffee just can't win and it's a loser for you.

Beverages that contain both caffeine and sugar, such as energy drinks and soft drinks, are the equivalent of a hurricane or tsunami in your system. Sugar in these drinks alone causes metabolic disturbances visible in the blood via the lipid, amino acid and energy related metabolites, and increases blood sugar levels up to three hours after consumption.

When compounded with caffeine, the effect became synergistically more noticeable[186]. Now we are talking like a meteor just hit the earth!

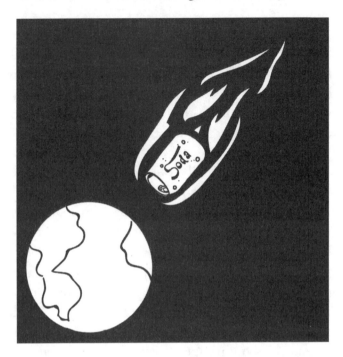

The bottom line is that even though there may be certain benefits in our present day stressed out systems, adding more confusion and stress via caffeine can just tip our body's balance over the edge. Why? Because the caffeine in coffee adds to our load of cortisol (the stress hormone) that is pumping through our veins and wreaking havoc in our bodies. You won't get the most benefits of the fast without dumping the coffee. Dump it, you won't regret it.

If you plan on cheating - I can already read your mind!

I am no fool! I know you. I have worked with patients long enough to know that coffee is one of the major addictions in life and for patients, one of the hardest habits to kick. I know you feel that you really need it, but just keep an open mind and don't commit to that thought process.

Take the road less traveled and give green tea a try. You will just have to bear through getting adjusted to the taste. After a while, you will see how you feel so much better with green tea as opposed to coffee and how you start to truly appreciate the taste.

Can "**Bulletproofing**" your coffee be the answer? This is coffee that has been popularized to be used during fasting and is blended with coconut oil and butter. It has been reported to be the panacea of health benefits for those aiming to live a healthy lifestyle, according to biohacker Dave Asprey, author of The Bulletproof Diet[187], a diet developed to enhance cleansing, health and mental clarity. The texture created by blending the coffee with those two ingredients makes it feel like it has thick and delicious cream in it. According to Dr. Andrew Weil MD, it is a much better fat to add to coffee instead of dairy[188].

There is much popular thought, but remember popular doesn't always mean right, as to what the benefits are. Firstly, because of the "healthy" fat added to the coffee, it improves the permeability of the cell membrane to absorb and bring the caffeine into the cell. Once inside the cell the caffeine can speed up metabolism. Caffeine brought into the cell may reduce the cortisol produced by the caffeine in coffee on the body. Thirdly, an improvement in mental clarity is reported.

So what's the real deal with creaming my coffee?!

What the research says is that while it is true that increasing lipids in your diet makes the cell membrane more permeable, the false claim is that the cortisol effect is blunted. In fact, the combination of cortisol, as stimulated naturally by the caffeine in coffee combined with high fat, is actually detrimental to our health. So the "Bulletproof Coffee" may not be the panacea that it is touted to be. It impacts the body causing insulin resistance, hyperglycemia and severe glycosuria[189] (blood sugar in our urine), the opposite effect of what you are looking for. Caffeine is known to help with mental clarity but this is old news[190] and the reason why many of us are hooked.

There is a lot of controversy with regards to coffee, some research supports its use and others not. Simply put, the effect of caffeine puts stress on our system. It improves mental clarity but it also contributes to leaky gut, bad gut bacteria, inflammation and stress to the D-Spot, which your body responds to by putting physiological padding of weight in the belly area in the form of water and excess fat. Dump the caffeinated drinks and dive into the green tea!

The following chart will give you a brief summation of the effects of different caffeinated beverages.

Phytochemical	Found In	Health Effects
Caffeine	• Coffee • Soft drinks • Energy drinks • Tea	• Hyperglycemia • Alertness
Caffeine plus sugar	• Coffee with added sugar • Soft drinks • Energy drinks • Tea with added suar	• **Major** hyperglycemia • Alertness
Caffeine plus fat	• Coffee with cream • Bulletproof coffee	• Hyperglycemia • Alertness • Insulin resistance • Glycosuria (sugar in the urine)
Caffeine with chlorogenic acid	• Coffee • Soft drinks • Energy drinks • Tea	• Hypoglycemia • Alertness • Inhibits receptors in the intestines that absorb • Leaves sugar in the intestines
Caffeine with theanine	• Tea	• Alertness • Increased focus • No hyper or hypoglycemia • Balanced energy • Balanced metabolism

Doesn't green tea have caffeine? So why is it allowed during fasting? Green tea has about three times less caffeine than coffee, but green tea has a special synergistic component known as L-Theanine.

The L-Theanine component of green tea has anti-stress effects[191]. It's actually used therapeutically to calm and relax the mind. So the effects of caffeine from green tea on the nervous system are therefore blunted.

In fact, one of the best things about green tea, and you will notice once you become a green tea connoisseur, is that it calms you down but keeps you alert and focused and able to concentrate on difficult tasks[192]. It's just incredible, and has benefits across the board and even for those who have hyperactive type disorders.

Your best option truly is GREEN TEA. It improves your metabolism vs. coffee and you are free to consume as much green tea as you like. One study reported a reduced risk in type 2 diabetes, with six cups of green tea vs. three cups of coffee[193]. A meta-analysis of green tea and green tea extract demonstrated that there was no negative effect on glycemic control, insulin or any of the laboratory markers related to diabetes with the consumption of green tea[194]. Another more recent meta-analysis supported this work, as well as providing a stable fasting blood insulin and in addition, reduced waistline circumference in type 2 diabetes patients[195].

The Goodness of Green Tea

How does that relate to us? During your fasting state, it will keep your blood sugar balanced and produce an improved metabolic profile[196]. Most of us have in some way shape or form a mild sugar dysregulation, and drinking green tea can help to keep us in a great spot. Super calm.

Of primary importance, is that green tea begins to help with healing the D-Spot lining and preventing negative changes in the gut environment as you're working towards healing. As you begin to include healthier fats into your diet and move toxins out of your body, without green tea you could experience an aggravation of a leaky gut, low grade inflammation and metabolic endotoxemia (toxicity from the inside). Green tea helps to negate these effects and in fact improves the D-Spot health, prevents dysbiosis[197] [198] and augments your cleansing.

Green tea also increases our bodies' natural antioxidants and master detoxifier agent glutathione[199a]. Glutathione is what keeps our bodies and livers clean, and there aren't too many things that help to support its production. An interesting fact is that we can measure the health of our glutathione and antioxidant status via the amount of hydrogen peroxide (H202) levels in the blood. One study done on pigs, that are of close genetic nature to humans and why we use pig insulin for diabetics, reported that increased intake of red cabbage and grape skins improved the levels of glutathione in the animals[199b]. We clearly don't want to eat a daily diet of grape skins and cabbage, so green tea can help in this area.

When you are fasting you are releasing toxins, so green tea will help to flush these out. Green tea is my absolute favourite prescription. However, there are a few things to be mindful of when selecting your green tea.

Sounds like a wonder drug to me. If you haven't been drinking the green tea, it's time to get on it, dunk it down your D-Spot and drop the other caffeinated beverages.

One thing to be aware of is that you must know where your green tea is sourced from as many can be toxic for different reasons. Some green teas are grown in soils that are toxic or laden with pesticides. As an example, green tea from China may be high in cadmium, especially those grown in the northwest part of the country as that soil tests for highest levels[200].

Green tea from Japan allows 50 ppm of neonicotinoid, a herbicide famous for killing off the bee population of the world and a strong neurological toxin to humans. That is much more than the allowable rate for fruit in Japan which is only 5 ppm[201]. You can imagine the multiplying effect if you are drinking a cup of green tea from Japan that contains 50 ppm of this neurological toxin 6-8 times per day. You don't need a calculator to know that this could become a problem.

Sometimes the issue exists that you simply do not know what you are getting in your cup of tea! Camelia sinesis is the species from which tea is made. Adulteration can occur with tea, by switching to a non-active species like Camelia pubicost[202] or other unknown herbs. One of the reasons I prefer loose leaf tea is you can see what kind of leaves you are getting. In a tea bag the leaves tend to be dried and could be mixed and old, adding rancidity to the problem. When consuming green tea for therapeutic benefit, quality really does matter.

Consume 6-8 cups per day for maximum benefit. Cold or warm, it does not matter. Make sure to consume before 4-5 pm, as there is caffeine and for those that are super sensitive, they may have an issue getting to sleep and that is not what we want. See what works for you. If you are super sensitive, stop sooner or reduce the amount of cups you're consuming.

I am a big fan of estate green tea. I try to avoid commercial brands and prefer loose green tea as the leaves are usually fresher. We work with our own sourced green tea, because I use it for therapeutic reasons with all of my patients, and I wouldn't want to negate the effects of green tea with the pesticides in many brands or any type of adulterations.

Troubleshooting With Green Tea

Nausea on an empty stomach? This is sometimes the first experience you may have had or are having with green tea. This is classically a sign of a very dysbiotic D-Spot, because the green tea begins to make the gut non-hospitable for the bad bugs. It is also a sign that you may have a high level of toxicity, the more bitter the green tea the more you will notice this because bitter mobilizes toxins out of your body.

How to reduce this problem: Dilute your green tea with water to make it less bitter. The other solution is to not over steep your tea. The longer that your tea steeps the more bitter it will become.

I'm a big fan of increasing the bitterness in the green tea, because bitters help to pump and dump the junk from your gall bladder into your D-Spot. This is the toxicity being processed and packaged to go out of your body through fat in the stools. Bile (which can be toxic) binds the fat in our diet. Bile is also self-healing for your intestines and they work interconnectedly. Healthy bile can alter the gut microbiota and the gut bugs can improve the health of the bile[203]. So if green tea begins to work on modifying the gut bacteria, this is just another way it contributes to helping heal your gut.

So if you must, start your tea practice with lightly steeped and begin to increase the bitterness as you go by steeping for longer. Aim to steep overnight and let the bitterness flow through your body!

Can't tolerate the caffeine in green tea? The other option to green tea is rooibos. Rooibos tea also helps with improving the amount of glutathione in our systems. It is detoxifying like green tea, in a different way without the caffeine.

Missing your caffeine kick? Go for Milky Oolong tea. A strong, rich form of Camelia sinensis that is partially fermented, where green tea is unfermented. The health benefits of oolong mimic green tea, assisting in weight loss, improving metabolic syndrome, ameliorating lipid and blood glucose profiles, anti-oxidative, protective for teeth and bones, and anti-bacterial[204].

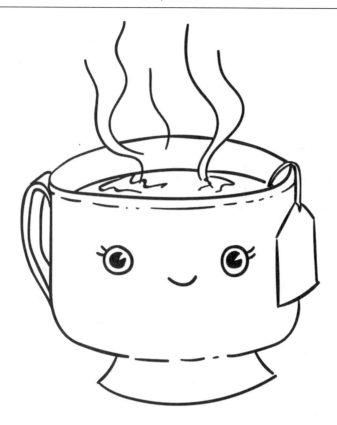

Plus it has more caffeine than green tea because of the fermentation process, so for those of you weaning off of coffee, oolong tea will become your best friend. I usually start the day with oolong and switch to green tea and then rooibos in the evening.

CHART OF CAFFEINE CONTENT OF COFFEE AND TEA[205]

Coffee Drinks	Size in oz. (mL)	Caffeine (mg)
Brewed	8 (237)	95-165
Brewed, decaf	8 (237)	2-5
Espresso	1 (30)	47-64
Espresso, decaf	1 (30)	0
Instant	8 (237)	63
Instant, decaf	8 (237)	2
Latte or mocha	8 (237)	63-126

Teas	Size in oz. (mL)	Caffeine (mg)
Brewed black	8 (237)	25-48
Brewed black, decaf	8 (237)	2-5
Brewed green	8 (237)	25-29
Ready-to-drink bottled	8 (237)	5-40

Fasting Do #2: Drop the Food, Do the Fat

During the fast, it is of utmost importance to avoid all proteins and carbohydrates. If you add these foods into your diet in the p.m. when you start your fast or in the a.m. while fasting, you will absolutely break the fast and unfortunately switch your metabolism back into burning carbohydrates. What you are looking for is to maintain fat burning mode for as long as possible so you can stay in the cleansing zone.

That means no fruit, vegetables, dairy, smoothies, juicing, broths with vegetables, proteins, nuts, seeds (except chia, see below). Consume nothing that contains carbohydrates or proteins as these are all considered foods.

For those of you starting and worried about not being able to maintain the 16 hours without any food, there are four choices to begin.

1. **Eat in the a.m. when you are hungry.** Instead of waiting the full 16 hours, just eat when you are hungry, and try every day to prolong the hunger sensation and fill up on your green tea. You will have to train your body to be without food. Be patient, eventually you will get there.

2. **Drink more fluids.** Many times our hunger is simply thirst. Water and green tea will fill you up and delay your hunger. Remember, feeling hungry is good and learning to listen to that signal is you getting in tune!

3. **Che, che, che, CHIA!** During your fast, to fill you up, take a teaspoon of chia seeds and soak them in 250 ml water for a few minutes, then gulp it down. This can help with binding of toxins that are coming out of the body as you fast. Chia seeds are full of soluble fiber. When soaked, they become a big glob that looks like mucus. Yes, I know, not very appetizing. This fiber is essential to bind and remove toxins. On top of it, the lipid profile of chia seeds also helps with reducing blood lipids[206]. All in all, a very good health tool.

4. **Use the Fasting Fat Bomb to get you through.** Fat bombs are allowed during the fast and won't break the fasting metabolism that you are trying to achieve. Actually it's quite the opposite, they will support and enhance it. A fat bomb can be as simple as downing a tablespoon of coconut oil or olive oil, or making Paleo Peppermint Bark. Fat will support your fat burning metabolism during the fast and keep you feeling full, so you want to keep these as fat based as possible.

Fat Bomb Recipes

Paleo Peppermint Bark: Blend softened coconut oil and mix in a few drops of peppermint essential oil. Pour onto a baking sheet and freeze overnight. Once frozen, break apart into pieces and keep frozen. Enjoy as needed. You may add some stevia for enhanced sweetness.

Coconut Oil & Vanilla Extract: Blend softened coconut oil and mix a few drops of vanilla essential oil. Pour onto a baking sheet and freeze overnight. Once frozen, break apart into pieces and keep frozen. Enjoy as needed. You may add some stevia for enhanced sweetness.

Fasting Do #3: First Fasting Supplements

Taking supplements is a true science. Timing is crucial. There are two very important supplements to start as you begin to practice fasting. Probiotics, and an alkalinizing agent.

These two supplements are important because they set the stage for the following steps in the D-Spot plan.

The right probiotics at the right time are a major key to health. So many people take any old random probiotic product and don't realize that each strain does something different and that you don't necessarily need an enormous amount, as long as you are optimizing how you take it and when. Many people take their probiotics religiously, however, they take them at the wrong time. Probiotics should always be taken on an empty stomach to prevent the stomach acid from killing off the good bugs. Here's how to enhance these first fasting supplements.

1. **Take your probiotics with green tea**. Another win for green tea! See, I told you this stuff rocks! It actually enhances the replication of good bacteria such as L. Acidophilus and L. Rhamnosus, two strains that are awesome for your gut. Since you are drinking green tea during your fast, this makes it the

optimum time to take your probiotics. Just make sure the tea water is lukewarm, - not too hot to destroy the good stuff.

2. **Take it with an alkalinizing agent.** Alkalinizing agents reduce stomach acidity and help gut bacteria to make its home in your D-Spot. Plus, alkalinizing also helps to reduce the acidity and inflammation in your body. Most are a combination of magnesium, calcium, potassium and bicarbonates. They are designed to support proper electrolyte balance that keeps the cells hydrated and nourished. This also facilitates nutrients moving in to your cells and toxins moving out of the body. Look for an alkalinizing agent that is sugar free and ideally made with non-GMO ingredients. Normally sold as a powder, alkalinizing agents can be mixed into any beverage, sports bottle or mixed with warm or cold water.

These are two key first fasting supplements to make sure all goes smooth and well. We will talk more about added supplementation in the section "Cleaning up your Supplement Regime."

Fasting Do #4: Fast Moves and Exercise in the A.M.

Some of the benefits of the fast you will be experiencing are a flatter stomach, weight loss, and feeling more focused in the morning. My favourite aspect about morning fasting is the fact that I feel so focused and unencumbered by food fog. I can do most of my genius work in the morning because my mind is so clear. I speed through what I need to do that demands a higher level of focus. One way that I have learned to enhance the fast is to add in exercise.

The optimal time to begin exercising is during the fast. When you are fasting and you infuse exercise in the a.m., you increase the amount of fat that is broken down and the benefits of the fast including the increased energy, focus, hormonal balance, immune regulation, cleansing, and weight loss.

Another important aspect is that exercise during the fasting state will help to reduce your hunger, will make you feel more satiated and full, as well as experience increased disciplined eating versus excessive indulgence[207]. All that from simply exercising during your fast. Let's say it together, "I can do that!"

Let's face it, exercise is crucial to health, we must have movement in our lives to be happy and healthy. You are aware that movement equals health. When we lose movement in our lives, we lose independence and we lose a part of ourselves. Movement brings us energy and vitality and keeps us flowing in the right direction. I always recommend to begin to add it into your life in whichever way possible.

Pepper exercise into your life like this:

- Take a walk after dinner.

- Dance as you clean the house, or just dance anytime.

- Take the stairs at work instead of the elevator.

- Park farther away with your car.

- Make outings based around exercise such as hiking.

There is always a way to increase the movement in your life. There is no excuse.

Many times what stops people from exercising is the fact that they believe they need to become slaves to the treadmill. Run for one hour in order to get a small benefit.

Many scientists and doctors like myself are recommending patients to do less for more benefit. Studies show that after just ten minutes of exercise, the natural hormonal surges that should happen with exercise, do. The benefit of the level is correlated with increasing intensity and increases over the time of the workout[208].

A little bit of cortisol is a good thing but becoming a slave to working out isn't healthy. When you go hard working out for hours and hours with a high intensity, instead of helping your body, you are doing quite the opposite. You are creating more stress for your system. You over do the amount of cortisol in your system.

Excessive increases in the amount of cortisol you create, and you start adding to the tire on your belly[209]. We get into the territory of diminishing returns for your investment in working out. This is why so many people lose their will power to work out. They slave drive themselves and are then victims of receiving negative benefits from all their hard work. Don't over do it.

When it comes to movement, it's important to season things with different forms of training. Moderate to high intensity training will increase serum cortisol whereas low intensity training decreases serum cortisol[210]. Variety and balance are keys to being healthy and getting the best return for all of the effort that you put forth.

One of the returns which I am all about is that if you are able to exercise during your fast, it can significantly enhance the speed at which your body is eliminating toxins because it increases fat oxidation[211].

Movement is part of a healthy lifestyle, but more importantly, for a healthy D-Spot. The big reason why, is that movement moves your inner organs, and naturally makes things move. If you are sedentary, nothing is moving and you and your D-Spot become stagnant. Regular movement is also incredibly important for the health of your D-Spot, in that movement can make movement happen (popping one out!).

Excessive training and dehydration will actually cause the opposite effect and choke the blood supply to your D-Spot[212]. Balance is key.

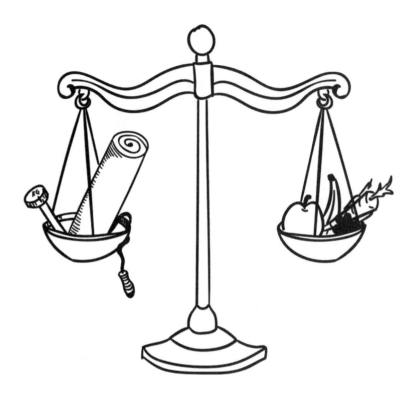

The reality is with exercise, less and more intense is best, seasoned with yoga to stretch and balance things out. My prescription is easy and executable, which is the most important part.

Ten to fifteen minutes three times a week of intense exercise really helps to get your system moving in the right direction and releases the toxins. My two favourite types of intense exercise are HIIT and Tabata training. You should also balance your routine with a yoga of your choice, three to four times a week, ideally in a hot room.

HIIT - High Intensity Interval Training - This is interval training where you exercise very intensely. It combines both cardiovascular aerobic exercise with periods of intense anaerobic exercise, similar to weight training. You do these short bursts of intense workout, then go to a rest phase and continue this pattern until you can no longer do it. It's intense, it works, and in general, you need less time on average to achieve your goals.

TABATA Training - This is a form of HIIT training, working out based on a clock timer - 20 seconds of intense working out, and 10 seconds of rest and relaxation. You can access a timer online at www. tabatatimer.com. I like Tabata because I feel it's very easy to do and you can do it with any random exercise that you have learned over the years, such as sit ups, push ups, jumping jacks, the dreaded burpees, and basically anything you know that you can do safely. Make sure that you are just intense for 20 seconds and then rest for 10. There have been times I have done this while making my lunch for work in the morning. Each Tabata is eight sessions of the 20 seconds work and 10 seconds relax, all done within a four minute interval. It's usually recommended to aim for at least twelve, which is three to four minute sessions. The way I look at it is four minutes is better than nothing. It gets your heart pumping, moves your lymphatic system and maybe gets you sweating a little and removing toxins.

Yoga - It will actually reduce the flowing cortisol in your system. It basically burns off the stress hormone cortisol. Research suggests that this is due to the alpha wave activation in the brain observed with a reduction of cortisol levels[213]. Alpha waves are normally secreted during wakeful relaxation with closed eyes. This is why I recommend mixing yoga into your routine three to four times a week, in between your HIIT workouts, so as to balance out your cortisol. This is also how we entrain our bodies for health by reducing the stress hormone and becoming more resilient to stress.

There are many forms of yoga. My favourites to recommend are those that are done in a hot room. This enhances your cleansing and sweating and the benefit that you achieve. Bikram is my favourite form which is very structured, using the same set of postures every time and the room is the hottest. Moksha is structured, but not to the same extent as Bikram, the room is less hot and the focus is more on the breath. Hatha, Kundalini and many other variations exist. The best thing to do is experiment and see which forms resonate with your body.

Because some people simply cannot exercise in the morning, and because of their daily life schedules, some people prefer to have breakfast and eat within 8 hours and then fast in the early part of the evening before going to bed and add their workout in then. This works just as well, but in my opinion, it may take more work to avoid the snacks before bed. But everything is doable if you put your mind to it!

Vitamin E with Green Tea Before Exercise

Another awesome tool to optimize and enhance the benefit is to make sure you load up on green tea before you exercise and supplement with vitamin E and EGCG, which is one of the active components in green tea. This is done to enhance your metabolic rate and burn more fat.

Your vitamin E supplement should contain a broad spectrum of vitamin E, including the alpha, beta, delta and gamma forms. If a supplement doesn't contain all of these forms you run the risk of depleting the others in your body. Your body requires all of them to function efficiently. Best to take in the morning during your fast, right before exercise.

Taking a green tea supplement which contains EGCG (an active component in green tea known as a catechin) is also super beneficial to take during your fast, before exercise with vitamin E. By this time, you either love green tea, or you aren't quite there yet and only able to consume one or two glasses per day. Adding in this supplement helps to augment the health effects of drinking green tea.

After Exercise, Support by Alkalinizing

Acid forms in our bodies with strenuous exercise, stress, as well as an unhealthy diet.

Simply by changing how you are eating, you will have begun to reduce the amount of acid forming in your body. This helps to enhance your exercise practice and we want to make sure you are getting the most out of your routine.

Alkalinizing the tissues pre and post workout helps to increase the amount of muscles that you build. As you well know, muscle is more metabolically active than fat tissue because it is more dense in terms of mitochondria which are the energy houses of the cells. So you look tighter and burn more calories, which are welcomed bonuses. Sweet! Beyond that, there are many health benefits, including helping your D-Spot become divine.

Alkalinizing also serves a very important function in your body. Enzymes, the key movers and shakers in your system which turn functions of the body on and off, can only work at a certain pH. If we are too acidic, typically they are not functioning properly. This is where alkalinizing plays such an important part in achieving overall health.

For the D-Spot, taking alkalinizing agents helps to alkalinize the tissues. Ironically, when you ingest an alkalinizing agent, it will temporarily alkalinize your stomach, only while you take it. Away from actively taking the dose, it actually helps to increase the acidity in your stomach. Remember, the ever important stomach acid is required to keep the entire digestive system in regulation of its pH. This function is of the utmost importance. Step one is changing the diet and step two is adding in those alkalinizers.

The other added bonus of alkalinizing is that it can improve your exercise routine. You know you are going to be sweating. Our bodies keep a tight regulation of important electrolytes. These electrolytes serve to keep your cell membrane potentials healthy, but also help with fluid transport between the membranes, keeping all the sections of your body in good shape. It prevents fluid retention and dehydration. It's part of optimizing the overall flow in your body.

Adding an alkalinizing agent into your daily routine will not only help with absorption of probiotics (when taken in combination), but will also help to enhance and support your muscles and tissues when you are exercising.

Break the Fast, Bring on the Feast!

Now is the time to finally break your morning fast. You drank the green tea and you've exercised as needed. Hallelujah! It's usually good to have somewhat of an idea for your meal composition between your lunch and dinner, or a proper plan such as the 7 Day D-Spot Meal Plan with recipes you can find at www.drmarisol.com. The way you start your day will be different depending on your life practice goals. However, the way that you end your day will always remain the same (in an ideal world, or at least during the program).

The most ideal first meal of the day truly depends on your goals. Most people will lose weight once they adopt the fast into their lives, but depending on how you begin your feast, will determine how quickly you lose the weight.

Now look, it is VERY important to be relaxed while you are eating. If you are stressed, your body is in the sympathetic, 'fight or flight' mode, and not the parasympathetic 'rest and digest' mode. One super simple way to ease your body into the parasympathetic state before each meal is to use the Queen of the Thrones™ **Grateful Dung™ Bracelet.** The Grateful Dung™ Bracelet is made with Tiger's Eye stones that serve as a guide to the healthy color of stools, as mentioned earlier. It also has a black obsidian, Swarovski crystal dung beetle bead. The dung beetle, or sacred scarab as it was called in Ancient Egypt, was worshipped as a symbol of rebirth and recreation of life. This beetle has the dirty job of rolling dung. According to Egyptian legend, this humble ritual serves to give life to the lotus flowers, the ultimate expression of regeneration. All of us are on a journey of constant rebirthing. As the sun rises and sets everyday, each day is an opportunity to be reborn.

To get your body into the parasympathetic state, ready to break your fast and receive the benefits of the healthy food to come, use this bracelet to do the **Grateful Dung™ Daily Dining Practice.** Here's how:

1. Hold onto the black obsidian, Swarovski crystal dung beetle bead

2. Name three things you are grateful for

3. Repeat this before every meal, and try to think of new things each time. As you do this it will become clear that there are many!

This simple yet effective gratitude practice can work wonders in your life, improving your digestion and contributing to overall happiness[214] [215].

Now that you know how to prepare yourself for breaking the fast, let's talk about the specifics.

The first meal of the day is very flexible. You can begin your day with a starchy carbohydrate heavy meal that includes the starches listed below, or follow the Queen of the Thrones™ Royal Feast Guidelines that include hearty protein, healthy fats, and heaps of vegetables. Or keep it simple and begin your feast with a smoothie.

Breaking the Fast Selections	Rate of Weight Loss
Starchy carbohydrate-based meal	Moderate
Hearty protein, healthy fats, heaps of vegetables — Royal Feast Guidelines	Moderate to fast
Royal Super Smoothie	Fast to super fast

The first meal of the day is ideal for a heavier, starchier meal. If you like to do vegetarian based meals of grains, legumes, nuts and seeds, this would be a good time for this vegetarian selection. Meals or snacks such as hummus and vegetables, hummus and crackers, beans and rice or any combination of the above would all be acceptable.

Examples of Starchy Carbohydrates	
Grains	Rice, wheat, quinoa, corn
Legumes	Beans, kidney beans, chickpeas
Root Vegetables	Potatoes, turnip, carrots, sweet potatoes, beets
Tuber Vegetables	Squashes, zucchini, pumpkin
Nuts & Seeds	Almonds, pecans, cashews

When you do these heavier starch combos, avoid adding in animal protein and too much fat. If you combine too much fat with starchy carbohydrates this is a recipe for weight gain. You can of course always add in more vegetables. You can't get enough of the goodness of those greens, yellows and reds!

That being said, if one of your major goals is to lose weight while improving your D-Spot, then the first meal of the day would be similar to the dinner meal. Break down of fat in the body occurs rapidly, the quicker that we achieve the fasting state. Clearly the easiest to digest foods are in the form of a smoothie, or to a lesser degree, a meal based on the Queen of the Thrones™ Royal Feast Guidelines. These meals keep our blood sugar regulated by reducing the amount of carbs in our system and can move us quickly into a fasting state.

A smoothie must contain protein and fat in order to keep blood sugars stable and keep you feeling satiated. A blood sugar regulation faux pas that is very common today is what people think of as the perfect smoothie, with protein powder and fruit. However, fruit mixed with a protein is a food combination that should always be avoided!

Everyone reaches for fruit or milk or yogurt when they make a smoothie. However, fruit and protein simply don't mix. It's very difficult for your body to be effective at clearing when there is fermentation happening in your stomach, because fruit requires alkalinity to digest and protein requires acidity of your stomach. The minute protein enters the gut, acid is commanded and the fruit just sits and ferments until the protein has passed and the environment becomes alkaline once again. So as you can see, a protein fruit smoothie isn't your best bet.

What you want to be putting into your smoothie:

1. **High protein** - A clean, good quality protein powder

2. **High fat** - Avocado, avocado oil, coconut, coconut oil, olive oil, nut butters

3. **Low glycemic index carbohydrate** - Organic spinach, kale, arugula, or a greens powder mix

4. **Fiber** - Freshly ground flax seeds (don't use chia seeds - remember, these are binders)

5. **Taste enhancers** - Cacao powder, ginger, cinnamon, vanilla extract

Royal Sup

Flavor
To taste:
- Sugar-free cocoa powder
- Cinnamon powder
- Ginger root

Greens
Unlimited:
- Arugula
- Broccoli sprouts
- Kale
- Spinach

Smoothie

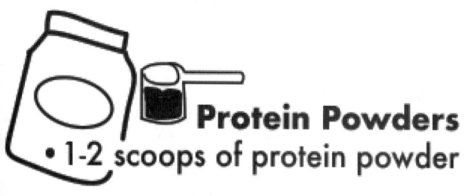

Protein Powders
- 1-2 scoops of protein powder

Healthy Fats
- 1/4 avocado
- 1-2 tbsp coconut oil
- 1-2 tbsp nut butter (almond, cashew, macadamia, or pumpkin seed)

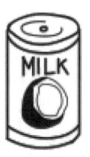

Liquids
- 1/2 cup of coconut milk
- As needed brewed organic green tea

It's best to structure your meal plans on a day to day basis, knowing what you will eat for lunch and dinner. The ideal is to ensure that by the time you are beginning your fast in the evening, you have more fat than carbohydrates in your D-Spot. This optimizes your digestion and cleansing mechanisms.

Between the Feasts

Sticking to two meals and avoiding snacking, just like your mommy told you, is the ideal. Your two feasts should keep you well satiated so that you don't feel the urge to snack. That is only if they have sufficient amounts of fat and the right foods to keep your blood sugar balanced. Those starchy carbohydrate meals that are allowed during the first feast tend to make you hungrier, leaving you wanting more in between meals.

When you listen to your body, and experiment with your food choices, you will see this to be true. Avoiding the snack, feeling hunger and feeling full are important to connect you to the timing of your body and how you are feeling. Remember, it's important for us to feel these sensations on a regular basis as they are how, we as humans, self-regulate.

However, due to very active lifestyles or strong healthy metabolisms, some people may choose to feed during the entire eight hours of the feasting time. Since we are all individuals, we must learn to listen for what is right for ourselves. Clearly, if you are an elite athlete training for more than 1 hour per day, you require increased caloric intake to have healthy reserves to be able to maintain your athletic performance.

If you are to snack, snack wisely and go for healthier options like nuts, seeds, protein smoothies or a piece of protein. Protein smoothies go a long way to helping you stay trim and rapidly achieve your health goal.

The Finish of the Feast

For the final meal of the day, how should you be feasting? Feasting with fat for the final stage of the day seems to be the best way you can go.

If you have a normal glucose tolerance you can consume a heavy carbohydrate meal in the p.m. without much effect. However, the reality is that both those with a normal glucose tolerance or impaired glucose tolerance do better with a high fat meal before bed and a carbohydrate based meal in the a.m[216].

Finishing the Feast	Rate of Weight Loss
Hearty protein, healthy fats, heaps of vegetables – Royal Feast Guidelines	Moderate to fast
Royal Super Smoothie	Fast to super fast

Protein Choices for your Fabulous Fasting Smoothies

When choosing a protein powder you want it to be clean, healthy, and easy to digest. For vegetarian protein, hypoallergenic pea, hemp or quinoa based formulas are great. If some liver-cleansing cruciferous vegetables or energy boosting nutrients like B vitamins are added, it's a bonus.

Beef protein isolate is another great choice for protein powder. Because it is animal protein, it is highly regenerating for muscles, tissues, and the immune system. Animal based proteins tend to have a richer texture than vegetarian proteins, which tend to be grainier or chalk-like in texture. I personally don't like whey protein, because lactose and casein are both common sensitivities for people.

Resetting Your Day Night Rhythm

So now that you are entraining your daytime feeding times, it's time to work at your night cycle. As I've spoken about in previous chapters, being in tune with our natural rhythm is essential to our health and especially to that of the D-Spot. Sleep has shown to reduce inflammation in gastrointestinal diseases[217]. This is always the first step that I work at with patients.

Sleep, Supreme Master Healer, Sweet Sleep

Sleep is the master calming agent of our bodies. Unfortunately, it's an area where most of you are suffering because insomnia, the lack of sleep, is an epidemic. We are so exposed to stressful stimulus daily, plus we surround ourselves with stimulus that upsets our natural rhythm, like wifi. How many cellular signals are you exposed to daily? Do you even know? You probably don't want to because those electromagnetic frequencies disturb your ability to shut down and turn off. Ironic, no? These electronic devices that so permeate our lives are culprits that affect our natural day and night rhythms.

It is important to have a good sleep and wake cycle, because this is what ultimately is the master of keeping your body healthy. You digest better when you sleep, you stress less when you sleep, your body detoxifies and cleanses when you sleep. When you get a good night's sleep you are less likely to over eat and to crave foods that would upset your D-Spot. One of the most important benefits is that good wake and sleep cycles reduce your risk of cancer. Many hormonal based cancers such as breast[218] and colon cancer are correlated to unhealthy regulation in circadian rhythms, basically the sleep and wake cycle.

How do you get your sleep back in shape in order to help with resetting your D-Spot? It's easy. Find out why your sleep cycle is off kilter. Typically, it's to do with a nutrient deficiency or excess, or external cues that are not conducive to a good sleep routine. Balance it out by supplementing that which is low and improving your nighttime routine with simple tools that promote awesome sleep.

First off, if you've implemented your exercise during the fasting period, you are already one step ahead of the rest because exercise can help to reset your day night rhythms, especially when practised in the daytime.

Many people either suffer from an inability to fall asleep or an inability to stay asleep. Sometimes too, that problem is compounded by anxiety and stressors of the day, that allow you to sleep, but it isn't an optimum and regenerative sleep.

The four types of sleepers are the following, and the issue is simply a deficiency in a natural hormone or neurological transmitter.

Sleeper Type #1: Can't Fall Asleep

You find yourself unable to go to bed at a decent time. You try to go to bed but you toss and turn, unable to fall asleep. Typically, this inability to fall asleep is due to a melatonin deficiency[219]. That deficiency can be caused due to excessive exposure to computer screens and blue lights. Blue spectrum light at night can inhibit our ability to produce our own natural melatonin.

Why is melatonin so important? It is a natural immune and hormonal modulator. Melatonin regulates our day night cycle and it is suppressed by blue light and all the technology that we use. Evidence suggests that melatonin in high levels in your body is protective against cancers, especially of the hormonal variety. People who have hormonal dysregulation problems tend to have big problems with keeping this neurotransmitter-like hormone at proper levels.

Melatonin is also a key deficiency in people who report having acid reflux, ulcers, problems with GERD and consequently with LES, the lower esophageal sphincter. If you have reflux, there is a link to having low melatonin. So it's essential to supplement in that case[220].

In addition, melatonin is known to help improve D-Spot motility at low doses, and at high doses it can slow it down. Yup, that's right, something that helps with sleep and hormonal regulation will help with the D-Spot being divine, no matter which side of the coin you fall[221]. It is no surprise that it is also beneficial to those with colon cancer, because they typically have very low levels. If you haven't noticed already there is a trend. Supplements and nutrients don't only work on one thing. They work in a variety of places in the body and you will notice the link between hormones, the nervous system and the D-Spot, so intimately intertwined, so synergistic.

Supplementing with melatonin starts at a dose as low as 3 mg, and can go as high as 20 mg (for many cancer patients, that is the goal). It is typically best to take melatonin about one hour before bed time. At lower doses, melatonin can help to improve gut motility and at higher doses melatonin will reduce gut motility.

One issue I have encountered personally and with patients, is that with melatonin you potentially could have nightmares. It is a rare side effect but I am one of those who experiences it. If this happens, typically melatonin supplementation is just not suited to you.

What's the alternative? To naturally boost melatonin, your best practice is to cut out all the blue light at night[222]. If you're unable to shut down all of your technology then your best option is to wear **blue light blocking glasses**. These typically come with an amber colored lens. I've had many patients benefit enormously from this simple change in lifestyle. Wear these glasses every night once the sun goes down[223].

Now my favourite, SUPER simple and highly effective way to naturally boost your body's melatonin is to wear an **eye mask** to bed. Simply wearing an eye mask supports our natural melatonin production without having to take a supplement[224]! I designed the Queen of the Thrones™ Beauty Sleep Eye Kit with this in mind. It includes an eye mask made with luxurious 85% organic cotton flannel to block out light and help you get your beauty sleep! It also comes with a 100ml bottle of 100% pure, certified organic, cold-pressed and hexane-free Cosmetic Castor Oil and a double ended eyelash and eyebrow applicator brush. Castor oil is excellent at nourishing the delicate skin around the eyes, preventing collagen loss and improving fine lines and wrinkles. It's also been used for centuries by Ancient Egyptians and Mediterranean Goddesses for long luscious eyelash growth and thick, beautiful brows. So not only does this kit help to increase melatonin production, it also provides amazing anti-aging benefits for the eyes. To get yours visit www.drmarisol.com.

Sleeper Type #2: Can't Stay Asleep

When you peacefully drift off to bed and then awaken in the middle of the night, it could be caused by one of a few things.

1. Overgrowth of Yeast

This will cause you to awaken in the middle of the night and urinate. This is due to the overgrowth of yeast irritating the mucosal wall of the bladder and ureter. The irritation makes you feel like you have to pee. This is very common as we age, since urinary tract infections increase with hormonal dysregulation and as women transition into menopause.

To help deal with this situation the best way to go about it is to do the D-Spot Meal Practice and follow the 3 step approach to healing your gut outlined in this book. Another key component is making sure to take a good quality probiotic. However, you won't get to the root of the problem by simply supplementing, you must complete the entire protocol to get rid of yeasts in the body.

2. Lack of Magnesium

Magnesium maintains the integrity of the bladder. With low levels of magnesium you will have the urge to urinate. With sufficient levels of magnesium in your body you won't have the excessive urge. If you are waking up because you need to urinate, a deficiency in magnesium could be the cause, but you still can't rule out the overgrowth of yeast (it could be a combination).

Magnesium has an incredibly powerful effect on relaxing the entire body. I like to think of it as the nutrient that relaxes the muscles and the mind, and makes your D-Spot move. Magnesium is one of the most important nutrients, and for women, one of the biggest deficiencies. Not only does magnesium work the magic as mentioned above but it is intricately involved in detoxification of excess hormones such as estrogen. It also feeds and supports the adrenal glands. It's typically one of the top prescriptions in my practice and I personally take it regularly for maintenance of good health.

3. GABA Deficient

If you can't stay asleep, the problem could be that your GABA (gamma-aminobutyric acid) levels are low. Stimulating your GABA receptors will help you maintain your sleep. It can actually counteract the effects of caffeine insomnia[225]. If you wake up in the middle of the night, you need to inquire if this is a problem. Typically, you won't be waking because you have to pee, you will just wake up because you are restless. This underrated neurotransmitter is also a staple in my practice. GABA is what puts our brains into the relaxed state.

Important to note, there are many things that can make us feel as though we have low GABA. Certain substances artificially augment our GABA. When these substances are withdrawn, we feel as though we are depleted in GABA, even though relatively, we are not. The substances that cause this include drugs of the gabaminergic kind, like benzodiazepines as well as alcohol and marijuana[226]. Excess stress, weak protein absorption and deficiencies in both magnesium and B6 can also do the same.

So your GABA can get low without you even knowing it. Your only clues will be difficulty with maintaining your sleep as well as less resilience to stress, which could present itself as anxiety or depression[227].

What blows my mind, is that besides supplementation, an easy way to augment the total circulating pools of GABA in your brain is to do consistent exercise over a long period of time[228]. This is one of the reasons we recommend to exercise during your morning fast! *Oh, Sh*t!* Now you know you gotta do it.

Please note that a deficiency in magnesium can cause a low production of GABA, which can mean that you may have symptoms of urinating at night as well. Sometimes it can be difficult to differentiate between these, in which case we treat for deficiencies of both. I always consider what the daily patterns are and if there is a lot of stress and sleep disturbances, I indicate both GABA and magnesium. Interestingly, women who have high levels of estrogen hormones, will have low levels of GABA. Why? Simply because women tend to have depleted magnesium, the higher their estrogen is. Consequently, the body will produce less GABA[229].

Like melatonin, GABA also has a protective effect on the gastric mucosal cells, especially against alcohol induced stress. It helps to maintain a healthy oxidative status and reduces ulceration of the stomach lining[230]. Not only is it helping to relax you and your D-Spot, but it is also helping to heal it.

To help with sleep, it's best to take GABA before bed. Should you wake up, you can take it to get back to sleep. You can also take it during the day if you are feeling more anxious or stressed out than normal. At bedtime and during the evening, the max dose is 500 mg. During the day you can take it much higher, up to 800 mg.

Another health hack to increase GABA is the Queen of the Thrones™ castor oil pack. This ancestral practice is a must-do to encourage calm, relaxation, great sleep, and to build your GABA and reduce magnesium spoilage, ultimately helping you poop. Do them every night for best results.

Sleeper Type #3: Tired but Wired

You're the type that is so exhausted, yet you go to bed and toss and turn all night. Your adrenal glands are typically burnt out at this stage. Your day and night rhythm needs a lot of work to repair. Working with adrenal adaptogens that contain herbs and glandulars can help to balance your day night cycle properly.

Glandulars of the adrenal gland can help stimulate natural cortisol when taken in the morning. In the evening, herbs are more effective at reducing cortisol. This serves to help you calmly move into the evening hours and reduce the increasing cortisol and stress hormones that may keep you up at night and upset your natural rhythm.

You need the rise in cortisol on waking for your body to work well, and then you need a decrease in cortisol in the evening to maintain good balance.

Herbs and glandulars are known to improve dysregulation of the adrenal glands and consequently can improve all aspects of life[231]. When the adrenals are off kilter, this leads to problems with your thyroid function. A common condition like hypothyroid also affects your D-Spot and one of the main symptoms is constipation. Our bodies are so interconnected!

If you focus on regulating your sleep wake cycle, this can change your life in a very positive way. It changes your mind, how you feel and how you react to stress. There are many benefits.

Sleeper Type #4: Overall Anxious

You are the type that tends to feel sensation in your body, tingling in your extremities and pounding in your chest. Overall, you need to learn to manage anxiety. Magnesium threonate or magnesium glycinate will be your best tools.

Whenever you take magnesium, it is ideal to add your alkalinizing agent. The potassium in an alkalinizing formula improves the functionality of magnesium. Plus, there is research that also suggests that potassium helps with sleep quality[232].

If you see yourself as one of these four sleeper types, it's imperative to take steps to improve your sleep patterns. It is usually the first thing I address with patients. Which one are you? Can't fall asleep, can't stay asleep, tired but wired, or overall anxious?

When you are aware and know what you are dealing with, **you can change your life.** Besides supplementation, there are very important and simple practices that will help you fix your sleep. Let's look into these now.

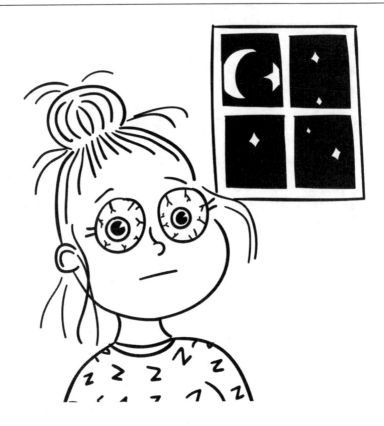

A Sound Sleep Environment

Not only do you need to work on reducing stress to achieve your best day and night cycle, but your environment needs to be conducive to the best sleep possible.

The Wifi Wean

Do you know that we are overexposed to dirty electricity and way too much wifi? This is one of the causes of many diseases. There is a possible link between "electrosmog", vitamin D deficiency and autoimmune diseases[233]. People are becoming more aware and researchers are starting to investigate something that naturopaths know; that we are sensitive to the frequencies emitted by all of our devices[234]. If brain tumours are associated with use of cellular phones[235], why wouldn't these electrical signals mess with our brain's sleep waves and affect our sleep? With everyone carrying around cell phones, and each of us outfitting our houses with wifi so we can constantly Google, Facebook and numerous other adventures in the world of the web, there has to be an impact on our lives and most importantly our regenerative sleep.

If we are trying to fix our sleep we must also address the physical irritants that are in our environment because they impact our inner world. The evidence is clear that these frequencies affect our bodies' ability to properly produce melatonin, it's not clear if that is the reason we are dealing with increasing rates of cancer. The low melatonin therefore has an impact on our natural circadian rhythm[236], something we must improve in order to balance the D-Spot.

Turn off the wifi on your phones before bed, there is no need to have them on. For those who are on call or that may need their phones, don't put it next to your bed, but as far away as you can from your head, where you can hear it. Put your home wifi on a timer, so that it shuts down automatically and this way you do not forget. Ours at home turns off at 10 p.m. and then starts again at 7 a.m. That way when we use it we have it available. Make sure to also put all of your phones on airplane mode and that way you avoid the exposure from your phone, but can still use your alarm clock.

Fit Bits and Self Tracking Devices

As much as I'm a fan of tracking and measuring how well you are doing in terms of taking steps in a day and finding out how many times you wake up during the night, there is a problem. These forms of technology are emitting electromagnetic frequencies that affect how your body is working. My suggestion is to try to find an app or use a good old fashioned pen and paper to track things instead.

LIGHTS OUT!

Blue and white light can brighten our lives and give us a burst of feel good hormones and help to cut our seasonal affective disorder[237]. The only problem is that the exposure all day and into the night can offset our natural biological rhythms as we discussed before. You need to turn off the blue light at least two to three hours before bed. For most of us this is impossible, because we are working late into the night on your computer, watching TV before you go to bed, or on your cell phone, iPad or other portable device that keeps you connected. It keeps you connected alright, to an unbalanced body system and sleepless nights.

To prevent this, shut off the lights! The other option is to use orange colored blue-blocking glasses in the evening like I mentioned before[238]. Yup, orange colored glasses, sexy don't you think?!

These glasses help to block out the blue light that stops the production of melatonin. With the orange colored glasses your melatonin can build, augment and improve your sleep, and remember, melatonin is one of the top anti-cancer agents in the body!

The other, easier way to do this, is to turn all the lights and technology off. Yes, you can, you can do anything you put your mind to. You need time to unwind as well.

Don't forget, it's all light. Even the light shining in from the street can affect your sleep, so blackout curtains are another way to make your sleep rock. Simply wearing an eye mask to bed, like the organic cotton eye mask included in the Queen of the Thrones™ Beauty Sleep Eye Kit, is another excellent way to block out the light and promote melatonin production[239].

Room Temperature

This is incredibly important. The room needs to be a few degrees lower at night, once again for the purpose of mimicking mother nature's natural rhythm, the nightly change in temperature. A room that is too hot will leave you restless and not allow you to delve into deep sleep[240].

Program your home temperature a few degrees lower at night to help you get that great restful sleep.

Castor Oil Packs

To get the maximum benefit of your castor oil pack practice, wear it overnight. The castor oil pack helps ease your body into the relaxed state[241] [242], preparing it for an amazing sleep. Our body is also doing internal clean up while we sleep, and castor oil packs help to enhance this by improving glutathione levels[243], reducing inflammation[244], improving smooth muscle function[245] and supporting a balanced microbiome[246] [247]. If you don't do any of the other things mentioned in this sleep section, I urge you to do this. Not only do the packs enhance your sleep, but they do so many other beneficial things for your body and feel oh so comforting, just like a big hug. They are my #1 prescription to all of my patients. I mostly love them because they support great paleo poops!

Journal

Before bed, to calm your mind, journal your day as well as what is left to do tomorrow. Write down your list and any ideas that you may have as they pop up. These ideas are at times amazing but can excite you to the point of preventing sleep. Other thoughts that might be disturbing should be written down and left in your journal as you close its pages. Writing your thoughts down can be one of the best ways to get them off of your shoulders, so to say. Responsibilities and the heavy weight of the day belong in your journal, while you wander into the clouds of dreamland.

I also recommend you write down three things that you are grateful for. Or use the Grateful Dung™ Bracelet. Be grateful for your daily grind. Studies show that gratitude practices can help promote long-lasting benefits for your mind and happiness[248] [249].

Routine

Regulation of the sleep cycle is benefitted by creating a "bedtime" routine within the ideal environment that you have created for your super sleep. You want to create a pattern over time and with repetition and practice, your body will recognize the signals to shut things down and begin to drift off into sweet sleep[250].

Washing your face, brushing your teeth, going to the bathroom, putting on your castor oil pack and eye mask, fluffing your pillow, writing in your journal, even getting frisky under the covers with your partner… as long as you do it in the same order frequently, the routine can help train your body to get a better night's sleep.

What's your sleep routine? _____

_____

_____

_____

_____

Commit to it every night.

Next Steps

Now that you've completed the first step and you are working at mastering the Connect phase, it is time for you to transition into the Clean phase. Remember, this information is not meant to treat, cure or prevent any disease. Always check with your doctor before beginning a new health plan.

CHAPTER 7

CLEAN LIKE A QUEEN

The Clean phase is where we get really serious about cleaning up the D-Spot. What you put into the D-Spot is as important as when you put it in. I want you to focus on putting clean foodstuff into your body, on multiple levels. This phase can also be very individualized for each person, because although certain foods may be considered healthy, it doesn't necessarily mean it is healthy for you. My healthy and your healthy can be two very different things. So let's find out what works for our bodies, so we can be royally Clean like a Queen!

Our focus in this chapter will be on:

1. Cleaning up what comes in

2. Cooking right

3. Consuming - your two week D-Spot Meal Practice plan

I also recommend that the Clean phase go in conjunction with the Calm phase for maximum benefit. So without much more preamble, let's get dirty! Oh, Sh*t!

Wash the crap away! Off your food, that is!

Food needs to be washed and cleaned as it is a source of bacteria and sometimes harmful chemicals like pesticides. The popular thing to say these days is 'eat dirt.' That's only as good as you knowing how healthy the dirt is that you may be eating, as in, does that dirt have good bacteria and is the dirt free of pesticides? Besides the dirt, there are many factors, including how the food has been stored and transferred, which will dictate how loaded the food is. So how do you get your food clean?

Storage: Many times, food has been stowed away in sheds for months at a time before it even gets to your kitchen pantry, especially foods like grains, legumes, nuts and seeds. These sheds may be humid, wonderful areas to grow molds of all types. These molds and yeasts consumed in your food will corrupt your D-Spot as it reinforces an environment for bad bugs to flourish.

How do I know this? I experienced it, when I lived in Nicaragua. I lived there for one month on a medical brigade. I lived with rice and bean farmers and I saw the practices of collecting and storing the crop.

Transportation: Our produce is transported in barrels and crates that are not labeled as organic only containers, which means that produce that has been sprayed can be carried in containers of organic foods that have not been sprayed. As a result, there is cross contamination. This contamination will mean more unwanted junk in your food.

So what can we do since we really have no control over how it is transported and stored? The following measures can help you reduce what will come into your system through polluted produce!

1. **Wash all of your food** - Washing alone is one of the best ways to reduce overall load of pesticides on your food. Don't skip this important step for it's important to your health[251]!

2. **Peel your fruits and vegetables if you can** - Peeling on its own can reduce the surface level of bad bacteria as well as pesticides. Of course you can't do this with leafy vegetables or soft skin fruit like strawberries, but you can sure do it with cucumbers and apples!

3. **When in doubt, scrub** - Again, not usable with all fruits and vegetables but you can do this with many. This removes the layer of toxicity on the vegetables.

4. **Soak or spray with our alkaline Free Your Food Solution**. Alkaline water is effective at eliminating a large majority of pesticides on produce and hydrogen peroxide is antibacterial and anti-mold/yeast.

How to make a **Free Your Food Solution:**

Soak

- Mix 250ml of water

- Hydrogen Peroxide 3% solution 5 drops

- 2 tsp. of baking soda

- 1/2 tsp. of Himalayan salt

  Mix ingredients together and soak your vegetables, fruits, legumes, grains, nuts and seeds for five minutes after washing them.

Spray

- Place mixture in a spray bottle.

- Spray on all of your vegetables, fruits, legumes, grains, nuts and seeds, then rinse or soak.

The soaking does have a better effect simply because there is more face time with the solution and the outside of the food. You can actually see the water get cloudy and sometimes change color.

Some people prefer to spray with a mixture of **vinegar** and water. However, in this phase of healing our D-Spot, we clean the diet further and fermented foods should be removed for a time. Therefore, the better option is to use the alkaline food wash. We don't want to introduce fermented products like vinegar as a cleaning agent quite yet.

Organic vs. Conventional vs. Local - Which is Best?

There is a lot of confusion about local, organic or conventional. What is the best option and bang for your buck?

Truly, it comes down to knowing not only what the label says, but having an idea of how the countries that are producing the organic food are operating. Organics from many Central American countries are labeled as organic, but I wouldn't stake my life on it. I'm not saying that they are lying as to the claim, however, many of these countries in Central and South America use banned pesticides known as organochlorines, such as DDT, in their non-organic crops. There is run off into the water supply that then may feed the organic foods[252], so you get much more than what you pay for.

Things to consider in your choice:

1. **How far is the food travelling?** The farther distance that a food travels reduces the amount of nutrients that are available to you upon eating. Also, produce is often picked green, and is not allowed to ripen naturally to get all of its goodness.

2. **What country is producing the organic food?** What are the conventional pesticides that they use? Do they use banned substances? Are they closer to the north and south poles? There is increasing toxicity in their atmospheres, as you move closer to the poles, due to the trade winds transporting toxicants to these areas of the world.

Here's my rule of thumb for organic, local and conventional (listed from best to least ideal):

1. **Organic local**

2. **Organic North American**

3. **Organic European Union**

4. **Organic Australian**

5. **Organic Latin American or local non-organic**

6. **Non-organic**

When in doubt, go to the EWG website. The Environmental Working Group is a non-profit organization that annually tests levels of pesticides in common produce. You can download their Clean Fifteen and Dirty Dozen lists as guides to help you decide which items should be bought organic. This is a good start as you clean up your diet if you can't find (or afford) 100% organic. The Dirty Dozen should be respected, and are the foods that no matter what, come hell or high water, you buy and consume these organic.

Food Sensitivities - Test or Trial

At this point in our plan we recommend that you seek out a naturopath who can test your food sensitivities via blood test. There are many tests out there but the best is to go to a qualified naturopathic doctor. We like to test IgG and IgE[253] as well as IgA on certain occasions, using the Elisa method[254]. The food allergy testing, in effect, ends up giving a real time view of what your immune system is doing right now and how it is responding to different "food" stressors that may be affecting your D-Spot. IgG testing has proven to be very beneficial to reduce the symptoms of IBS[255] [256]. Check out the link to Your Lab Work website on the resource page at the back of this book for a lab that I use and trust to get this testing done.

I always emphasize to patients that the test, like all testing, must be repeated and it is not perfect. It is in repeating the test that you see your true food allergies and/or exposure sensitivities. The exposure sensitivities change over time as you decrease your exposure to them. Only if the food is a TRUE allergen, will it remain a constant from test to test, no matter how much or how little the exposure. It is in my opinion one of the most valuable tests that someone can do. When we work on cleaning up the D-Spot, one of the first steps is to clean up one of the biggest promoters of irritation, the food you eat all day long.

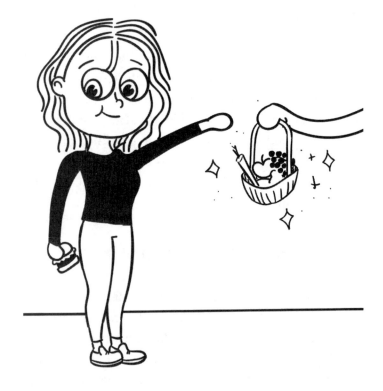

Why is the testing not perfect? Because no testing is; you still need a clinician to interpret your problems and issues in the context of the testing. Algorithms to help with long term treatment and management are incredibly important[257].

When unable to test, an elimination diet is the gold standard[258] to deduce food sensitivities. However, it is based on objective symptoms and the problem with this is it takes a long time to accomplish and a very restrictive diet must be followed. Many food sensitivities can take up to 72 hours to show their symptoms, so often times it can be hard to say, "Hey, that sandwich I ate 72 hours ago made me get this headache today." Hmm, what are your thoughts? Not the easiest way to go about it, for sure.

If you are to do this method, we recommend removing the foods that come up most frequently in testing as listed below.

- Dairy - all forms cheese, yogurt, ice cream, milk

- Gluten and wheat

- Legumes

- Nuts

- Corn

- Grains - rice, amaranth, millet, oats

- Potatoes

- Strawberries

- Eggs - typically egg white, but removal of all is best

- Beef

- Pork

- Tuna

For a period of two to three weeks these foods are completely removed from the diet as part of the Clean phase. You must be very careful to look at all ingredient lists, because many of these can sneak into your foods without you knowing. After the clean out period has finished, one by one you begin to reintroduce the foods in a specific manner.

As an example, you introduce wheat back into your diet. On day one, you have wheat and wheat products at each meal for the first day. Then stop the food for the next two days. Watch and record your symptoms. Do you get moody? Do you have a belly ache? Do you simply not feel right?

Sometimes the symptoms are loud and clear and at other times they can be quite obscure. The reason to wash out and not eat them for two days is you don't want to have too much of that one food type in your system, because your body can start to blunt the symptoms, almost a numbing, so to say, to the symptoms caused by the food. If after three days (72 hours) you have no symptoms, the food is free from sensitivity for you. Now you move on to the next food, repeating the exact same process.

As you can imagine, it takes a long time to get through all the foods. However, the result is worth it! So if you're up to it, and you can't get testing, then this is what I recommend. Here's one word of caution: some people may have random allergies to healthy foods that they wouldn't realize, because it isn't a common food sensitivity, so it isn't excluded during the elimination diet. This is where we find the food sensitivity testing to be essential and much easier.

So if you complete an elimination diet and you still don't feel the best, it may be because you are one of those, like I was, that had random food sensitivities outside of the common ones.

Fortunately for you, the D-Spot Meal Practice omits most of the common food sensitivities. If you haven't had food sensitivity testing done, at the end of the two week Clean you can introduce the foods as mentioned above and try to determine your own sensitivities.

Food Intolerance

If you know you have food intolerances to dairy or other foods, avoid them during the Clean phase. Remember, food intolerance is typically a lack of an enzyme to be able to digest the food, so this can seriously aggravate the D-Spot.

COOK!

During the Clean phase, your options for food ingredients are going to be reduced. However, that doesn't mean that your meals have to be boring or bland! It's time to bring on creativity in your food preparation. The biggest issue, I find, is people think that food preparation needs to be difficult. The reality is, it truly is simple and it's just about getting back to basics.

Cooking your food is of the utmost importance when dealing with an irritable bowel. Often times people recommend to eat raw for health promotion. Raw is, in my opinion, difficult for people with an irritable bowel. The exception is raw vegetables that are dry and easy to digest, like organic salads that aren't thick or rough. During the Clean phase, most meals will be either lightly cooked, steamed or one pots. Raw vegetables are kept to a minimum.

Boil: Boiling is a quick and easy way to get your foods cooked. After boiling, keep the fluids, since they are rich in nutrients and can be used as a base for soup. Please make sure to always wash and rinse your vegetables before boiling to remove any contaminants.

Steam: This is the best option for cooking to preserve the nutrients in the food. It also seems to be the fastest. I know that I can steam a head of broccoli to perfection in less than five minutes if the water is boiled beforehand.

Bake: Baking can make your life easier because it's possible to make your entire meal at the same time. For example, you can put a chicken into the oven with whole onions and veggies on the side. It speeds up your time in the kitchen, giving you more time to food prep or time to spend with your family, while making dinner. Oh Sh*t, spare time!

Broil: Broiling your veggies is great if you want to seal in the flavour and spices and give them a nice golden color. Use coconut oil instead of butter to broil things like asparagus. Usually, broiling occurs at the end of cooking or baking of a vegetable.

Fry: Frying stands apart from other cooking methods, because it's always gotten a bad rap, but not from me! In my home, we cook with coconut oil and make things like stir-fries and eggs. There is no oxidation to the oil and therefore no deleterious health effects. The only problem is you have to like the taste of coconut. Many of my patients continue to fry with olive oil because of a taste aversion to coconut. But be forewarned, olive oil does not have a high heat tolerance and will oxidize and become a trans-fat, and we all know that is not healthy for us.

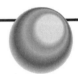

PEARL OF WISDOM

If you haven't heard what a trans fat is, then you've probably been living under a rock for the past decade or so. Trans fats are dangerous to your health. They are a byproduct of manipulating & heating oils. They occur in oils that can't handle the heat of the kitchen. The best oils for cooking with high heat are coconut oil & avocado oil. Coconut oil is a saturated fat, so therefore, has no double bonds to be broken. Avocado oil has only a few, so it's less likely to become a trans fat. Remember, in my opinion, its always best to COOK WITH COCONUT!

One pots: These are by far my favourite in terms of time and ease. These are most useful in the fall and winter months, when the starchy vegetables are in season and easily available. Mix vegetables with a meat base and add in coconut oil and spices to taste. It makes an easy to digest meal because all of the flavours have blended together.

What to cook with

The most health promoting oils include coconut, avocado and olive. The best oil to cook with is coconut due to its ability to withstand high heat. Avocado oil can be used for cooking if needed, but is better used cold. Olive oil should be used cold.

Clean your diet

The Clean is simple and easy to follow. It's designed for the irritable bowel to remove the stressors that can insult the D-Spot, heal the gut lining and regulate digestive movements. Many diets have been studied with regards to irritable bowel and there seems not to be a consensus as to what is the best[259]. This diet is created from both my personal as well as clinical experience, and is the gold standard at my clinic, Sanas Health Practice.

The principles are simple, based on three food groups;

1. **Heaps of vegetables**

2. **Hearty proteins**

3. **Healthy fats**

These are the Sanas Health Practice food principles, much like the standard food pyramid, however, mine looks a lot different! We model it on what your standard plate, or "Royal Feast" should look like.

Royal Feast Guidelines

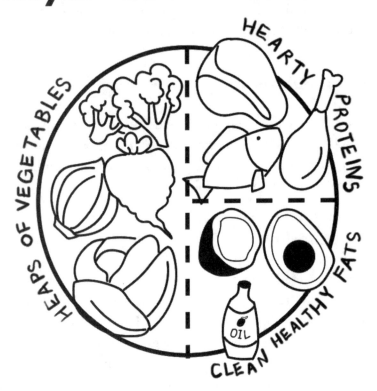

Fruits
Consume fruits sparingly as a snack & away from proteins.

Heaps of Vegetables
Enjoy at least a half a plate of colorful non-starchy vegetables. Raw, roasted, steamed, grilled or in a soup/stew.

Grains & Starches
Enjoy whole foods like quinoa in 1/2 cup servings/day. Limit starchy vegetables like corn & potatoes in addition to grains like rice & gluten-free pastas or bread.

Hydration
Drink 4-6 cups of organic green tea daily, in addition to water & herbal teas like rooibos for a total of about 2L per day.

Hearty Proteins
Enjoy lean & well-sourced animal proteins like eggs, fish, chicken, turkey, beef or game. Other proteins include hemp hearts, legumes, or protein powders.

Clean Healthy Fats
Enjoy plenty of whole food fats like avocado, walnuts, pumpkin seeds & coconut cream; in addition to oils like olive, avocado, & coconut.

Dairy & Alternatives
Enjoy alternative dairy like almond, cashew, or coconut milks. Consume dairy products like milk, cream, cheese, & yogurt sparingly, if at all, as they are inflammatory & often impair digestion.

Heaps of Vegetables - The largest portion of your royal feast should be a variety of healthy vegetables. Vegetables such as beets are my absolute favourite due to their nutrient content. Beets are a liver supporting, blood boosting and nitric oxide increasing vegetable[260]. Nitric oxide is a powerful molecule that heals the D-Spot[261]. Even though it's a starchy vegetable, it's so healthy for you, it's positives beet out the negatives (pun intended). Other favourites include red and green cabbage, broccoli, Brussels sprouts, asparagus, cauliflower, onion, garlic and all the leafy greens that you can find. Green is goodness and an essential element of being healthy.

Hearty Proteins - Lean meats, beef, fowl (chicken, turkey, quail), wild game, fish and seafood.

Healthy Fats - Oils can often carry high levels of toxicity so it is important to choose cold-pressed, non-refined and organic oils. Consuming significant amounts of healthy, clean fat helps to nourish your body and cells but also helps with cleaning up your body. Fat is a win-win situation. Remember, cook with coconut! **Avocado** and **olive oil** are best used 'All Over'. Other oils that I like and recommend to indulge in are hemp oil and pumpkin seed oil. However, these are not to cook with.

Oils are of such importance because they can act as carriers to help mobilize toxins and chemicals out of the body. They are also a powerful anti-inflammatory agent for your body and D-Spot. You always want to purchase oils 100% organic, in dark glass bottles (coconut oil is excepted as light will not damage it). Healthy oils bring goodness in and carry the garbage out.

Guidelines:

- For two weeks during the Clean phase, we cut all starches out of the diet. This includes all nuts, seeds, legumes and starchy vegetables like winter squashes and potatoes

- Avoid your food sensitivities and if you don't know them, avoid all the foods that are on the common allergens list

- The majority of vegetables should be cooked. Only use light, leafy raw vegetables.

- Onions/garlic/leeks - these sulfur containing vegetables can irritate the gut and must only be consumed cooked, in small amounts as seasoning

- No fermented foods

Heaps	Hearty	Healthy
Vegetables	**Wild Game**	**Fats**
• Beets	• Moose	• Olive oil
• Raddish	• Buffalo	• Avocado oil
• Red cabbage	• Bison	• Coconut oil
• Beet greens	• Deer	• Pumpkin oil
• Broccoli		(organic)
• Brussels sprouts	**Fish**	
• Kale	• Salmon	**Sweetener**
• Kohlrabi	• Sole	• Stevia
• Green cabbage	• Haddock	
• Swiss chard	• Halibut	**Non-Dairy Milk**
• Avocado	• Herring	• Coconut milk
• Green onion	• Anchovies	(in a can)
• Leeks	• Shrimp	
• Lettuce	• Lobster	**Seeds (soaked/**
• Arugula	• Crab	**freshly ground)**
• Asparagus		• Quinoa
• Celery	**Meat**	• Flax
• Summer squashes	• Turkey	• Chia
• Chayote	• Chicken	• Pumpkin
• Zucchini	• Beef	• Sesame
• Cucumber		• Sunflower
• Cilantro		• Almonds
• Parsley		
• Dill		
• Fennel		
• Green peppers		
Fruit		
• Lemons		
• Limes		
• Avocado		
• Coconut		

In this phase, your diet will be the focus and you will shift to a very nurturing food selection. Only foods that heal or regenerate are enjoyed. Nothing that causes irritation and nothing that has an excessive amount of sugar in the form of glucose and fructose for the body should be consumed. Simply real, fresh, whole foods!

How

Many foods, although 'healthy', actually feed the bad bugs in our gut or create quite a bit of irritation, making it a hospitable environment for the bad bacteria. When we eliminate those foods for a minimum period of two weeks, we can experience a great change in health, as well as healing of the D-Spot. The changes begin to occur within a twenty-four hour period. It's surprisingly that fast! We are superhuman after all. The longer you maintain this diet, the better in health you will be. So even though we suggest you follow it for only two weeks, you can challenge yourself to more. Or alternatively, if you find longer than two weeks to be too hard you can alternate, two weeks on, two weeks off. Figure out what works for you.

You will become more sensitive to the foods that aren't right for you. At first, this may seem like a bad thing, but in reality, it's the best thing that could happen because it means that your body can now feel when a food is negatively affecting your D-Spot. You will become in tune with your D-Spot, an absolutely incredible talent.

You have the ability to listen and use your intuition to understand what is actually good for you or not. Before this diet, you could eat bad food and it would not bug you, or at least you thought. In reality, you were so disconnected from your self and your body that you couldn't feel how food was affecting it. It is still affecting your body, probably not in a good way, but you just can't feel it if you aren't in tune with your D-Spot. Eating foods that you are sensitive to causes immense stress on your system and inflammation, silent inflammation, which is the 'silent killer'.

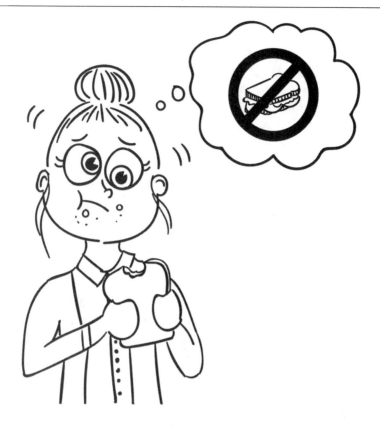

The "Somewhat Healthy Food" list that needs to be removed in the Clean phase

Starchy and Sweet Vegetables: Although vegetables, the list below includes vegetables that are high on the glycemic index. That means when you eat them, they have a large amount of sugar in them causing a spike in blood glucose levels. This promotes bad gut bacteria. They also put you on the roller coaster of insulin because of excess sugar content.

They include:

- Potatoes

- Corn

- Sweet potatoes

- Carrots

- Winter squashes

- Red peppers

- Tomatoes

- Rutabaga

- Turnip

Exception - BEETS! Although a sweet and starchy vegetable, this one is so packed with goodness and helps your liver detoxify, as well as clears out your D-Spot. Recent research demonstrated that modified beet pectin was effective in treating colon cancer cell lines and this effect was enhanced by alkalinization of the cells[262].

You simply cannot live without this one. It's a high source of glycine, an amino acid that stimulates detoxification, as well as a source of nitric oxide. Nitric oxide is the anti-aging drug. It is what is produced by viagra to help with erection; it keeps you young and going strong. Source it naturally and eat your beets, as much as you can, including the greens[263]. Castor oil packs are another source of nitric oxide[264 265], so important for our health.

Fermented Foods, Molds and High Histamine Foods

These foods often times are mistaken as very healthy foods, because they contain bacteria. Many people are mistakingly led to believe they will help to repopulate their good gut bacteria. They are very beneficial in a healthy gut but in a deranged D-Spot, these foods, along with leftovers that have sat too long, will stimulate the increase of histamine.

Histamine released in the body is what happens when you are exposed to poison ivy, or an anaphylactic allergy. You get hives and serious life-threatening inflammation. That is exactly the same process that occurs in the D-Spot when you eat fermented foods that contain histamine. If your D-Spot isn't healthy, it can't tolerate these types of foods. When your D-Spot is relatively healthy, the histamine that is produced from lactobacillus reuteri acts as a reducer of inflammation[266]. Fermented foods typically lack the reuteri genus of lactobacillus[267].

The other thing with fermented foods is that they increase biogenic amines such as tyramine and histamine. These wreak havoc on the D-Spot that is trying to become divine. These are majorly irritating to the body, and in some cases can be so toxic that there are reports of it killing people. Biogenic amines are created by the body. They are, in fact, many of the neurotransmitters that live in the brain, but too many external ones cause problems, histamine being a big culprit[268].

Fermented foods that are to be avoided in the Clean phase are:

- Vinegar

- Cheese

- Alcohol

- Pickles

- Olives

- Kombucha

- Sauerkraut

- Kefir

- Pickled beets

- Pickled eggs

Foods that are molds that should be avoided in the Clean phase are:

- Mushrooms of all types, i.e. button, portobello, cremini.

Foods that are high in histamine that should be avoided in the Clean phase are:

- Processed and cured meats - salami, ham, bologna, hot dogs.

- Leftovers that sit in the fridge for too long (more than a day) allow bacteria to grow and increase the histamine load

Note: Certain foods may have elevated levels of histamine and are still included in your foods to include lists, avocado and tea are examples. Although each is high in histamine, they are still used during the Clean phase because their health benefits outweigh the histamine effect.

Seeds, Grains and Nuts

Seeds, grains and nuts are all products of plants. The categorization can be confusing so here's a little clarity.

Grains: Now it's common knowledge that grains are inflammatory foods. Grains are seeds that come from grasses. **A few examples are:**

- Wheat

- Barley

- Malt

- Rice

- Rye

- Sorghum

- Triticale

- Spelt

- Millet

- Oats

Different components, like lectins, irritate the gut, create inflammation and are also found to be part of what causes allergic disease[269]. To heal the D-Spot we must reduce the amount of inflammation and inflammatory foods that enter gut. In addition, grains are generally high on the glycemic index, therefore spike your glucose and then insulin. They also have anti-nutrients such as phytic acid, which inhibits absorption of nutrients such as minerals and trace elements in the D-Spot[270 271 272 273]. So ideally, if we are trying to clean and heal the D-Spot, grains should be avoided. As you will note, they are not on the Clean food list.

Seeds: Certain seeds are super. Remember, they do not come from grasses. They are in a category of their own and we recommend these to be consumed wisely. Like grasses, they also contain anti-nutrient components such as phytic acid, however, not all in the same amount. Certain seeds have compounds that cancel out the anti-nutrient effect. **Here are the most commonly consumed seeds:**

- Flax seeds

- Chia seeds

- Sesame seeds

- Hemp hearts

- Pumpkin seeds

- Quinoa

- Amaranth

- Sorrel

- Buckwheat

- Almond

- Pine

My favourites of the above list include the following:

Quinoa is the queen! It is an ancient grain that provides good bacteria for the intestine, but also has the ability to degrade phytic acid. It truly is a super seed considered by many to be an excellent source of protein[274]. This is a key food on your plan.

Fill up on flax seed! Flax seeds are an excellent source of Omega 3's and potassium[275]. They're also a super rich source of lignans, which act as phytoestrogens, in its fiber/meal. Flax, having the highest amount of these, helps with the prevention of hormone dependent cancers such as breast, ovarian and prostate[276]. Plus, with the high quality fiber content, it helps with going to the bathroom too!

Say yes to sesame! This seed is known for its high levels of Omega 6 oils and dietary calcium[277]. But in addition to that, it also contains a lignan known as sesamin. This lignan has recently been shown to aid in the development of chondroitin sulfate, which is a proteoglycan or connective tissue component made by chondrocytes. These cells are incredibly important for bone sculpting and remodelling[278].

The power of pumpkin seeds! An excellent source of Omega 3 oils as well as zinc, these seeds taste delicious with anything you may add to them. They are a natural anti-microbial that will help with resetting the gut microbiome[279]. They also help to naturally improve your sleep and mood via the serotonin pathway, because pumpkin seeds contain high quantities of serotonin's precursor amino acid, tryptophan[280]. I love the taste and like to recommend it to men who have benign prostatic hyperplasia (BPA), because it's protective and also shows promise for hormonal based cancers of the prostate[281]. Pumpkin seed oil is also quite stable with heat, so it's one of the oils that we go gaga for[282]. With pumpkin and all gourds, you must ABSOLUTELY go organic because this plant accumulates more heavy metals from the soil than other plants[283 284].

Chia seed saavy! I love my chia seeds because they are the most amazing source of soluble fiber. Avoid chia with protein, but incorporate it into high carbohydrate meals such as vegetables only. This is because chia is incredible at slowing down the release of carbohydrates into the blood, much stronger than flax seed[285a], something that protein already does. Plus, the viscous fiber will bind to protein and take it out of the body, but protein is something that you desperately need to be absorbing. The biggest mistake is that many people put chia seeds into their protein smoothie. It's okay in a juice, on vegetables or a protein-free meal on pasta, but keep it away from the protein, please!

Always an almond! It's a seed not a nut, and with this seed you'd be hard pressed to find someone who doesn't find them delicious. The benefits are many, from containing high levels of calcium, to the oil acting as an anticancer agent in colon cancer[285b]. An extract from the skin of the almond is apparently beneficial in breaking down fat cells[286], heart disease and so much more. But it seems it's best to break down the nut, fresh, to release all of the many benefits.

Note: During the Clean phase, make sure to freshly grind all of your seeds before consuming them. Unground seeds can cause havoc on an irritable D-Spot. Post Clean, it can be hard to digest and extract all of the nutrients from the renowned seeds. Therefore, it's still highly recommended to grind them fresh, as it releases all the goodness of the seeds[287]. So blend 'em up before you enjoy.

NUTS about Nothing

Nuts are notorious for having molds growing on them. When you are trying to change your D-Spot from dysbiotic to divine, you need to reduce the amount of mold or mycotoxins that you ingest.

Pistachios, as an example, are quite high in mycotoxins, otherwise known as fungus. There are a variety of molds that can grow. Aspergillus flavus is one of the molds which create a toxic by-product known as aflatoxin. This toxin is a known carcinogen to humans and is strictly regulated to be below 4 ppm in the European community[288]. Pistachios that are in the shell and not open lack this mold. However, those that have the characteristics of being slightly opened and brown in color contain it. If the hull has split in the early phase of growth it will be more contaminated than the hull that has split later on in the stages of growth and cultivation[289]. Post harvest handling plays a big role in the nut mycoflora and therefore, for the consumer, post purchase handling is necessary for you as well[290].

Nuts have also been banned from schools all over North America for being a major food allergen. Not surprising, they also often come up in food sensitivity testing. If you haven't tested your sensitivities, we recommend to stay away from nuts as you simply never know whether you react to them or not. Nuts also contain the previously mentioned anti-nutrient phytic acid.

Now nuts are not all bad. They are a source of many healthy nutrients as well as phytochemicals[291]. Good healthy oils abound in nuts, and many of them simply taste great. Here are some of the most commonly loved nuts:

- Cashews

- Pistachios

- Hazelnuts

- Walnuts

- Chestnuts

- Brazil nuts

- Macadamia nuts

Leggo my Legumes

Everybody loves legumes, especially if you're aiming to go vegetarian or vegan. They are absolutely part of a healthy plant-based diet, that I hope includes some meat. But when you're working on the Clean phase, we have to leggo the legumes.

They are irritating to heal and hence, frequently come up on food sensitivity testing, especially navy beans and kidney beans. This is mainly due to the irritation from the skin of the legumes on the D-Spot. It's the lipopolysaccharide component of the skin, which can be beneficial to the immune system, but in an irritable D-Spot causes problems. Adzuki beans are an example. In mice, they have been shown to reduce inflammation in the colon by lowering certain markers of inflammation, like nitric oxide. This is good in the long term, however, in the short term while trying to fix an irritable bowel, nitric oxide is actually needed for the healing to happen because it increases blood flow to the area, protects the mucosal gut lining and maintains vascular flow[292]. Castor oil packs, if you recall, help with the release of nitric oxide to heal the gut. So we can use this as a strategy to long term care[293]. Make sure to do your castor oil packs everyday!

Other concerns, I will include as an example, the genetic modification of soy. Genetically modified foods are not properly recognized by our body. This is noted by the immune system responding differently to wild soy versus GMO soy[294a]. This may be a causative factor in changing our immune system responses as we still don't know enough about the effects of GMO foods on the body.

Of course, legumes also carry with them the potential for molds just like seeds and nuts with aspergillus flavus, the producer of aflatoxin. Peanuts have been notoriously branded as they are known carriers of aspergillus flavus and with that, the carcinogenic compound aflatoxin. List of common legumes:

- Navy beans

- Kidney beans

- Peanuts

- Soy beans

- Soy

- Lentils

- Chickpeas/garbanzos

- Adzuki

- Mung

- Peas

Lovers of lentils and purveyors of peas need not worry. Soon after the Clean phase you can re-introduce all these lovelies back into your health practice. They are delicious and offer many benefits, peas have been shown to be a strong anti-cancer food[294b]!

Anti-Nutrient Annihilation

Remember how we spoke about phytic acid? The anti-nutrient component of grains, seeds, nuts and legumes? There are ways you can reduce its effect and it is simple.

Soaking, sprouting and **roasting** are ways to take charge of this anti-nutrient[295].

Soaking will help with reducing the molds/mycotoxins on them (that's why you do the alkaline Free Your Food Wash).

Remember, they call **phytic acid** an anti-nutrient because it chelates, which means it binds to important minerals and robs your body of them. Minerals are required for all functions of our body. It also inhibits pepsin, which is required for breakdown of protein. Phytic acid is a sneaky opponent, hiding away in food that is also jam packed full of goodness.

So how do we mediate these two culprits, mold and phytic acid?

Soaking in the Free Your Food wash can do both. It reduces the mold/bacteria coming in on the nuts and stops phytic acid in its path.

Roasting will make it taste yummy and inhibit phytic acid from binding to your minerals and proteins.

Sprouting can also help deactivate the phytic acid, one of the reasons why sprouted seeds are a lot easier to digest. In addition, the bonus is that sprouted seeds tend to have increased nourishment[296]. Sprouting can be as easy as soaking a paper towel with water, placing it on a cookie tray or sheet and placing the seeds and nuts on the tray in the sun. Leave for a few days and voila, a new type of crunch for your salad.

Fruits

Why are there barely any fruit on the clean foods list? The answer is that many fruits are made up of a component known as fructose, a naturally occurring form of glucose. These are short chain carbohydrates that are notorious irritants of the D-Spot and also feed bad bugs that live there. For a period of time, we need to let these go. Not forever, but just until we can get some D-Spot balance. This is an approach similar to that taken by the FODMAP diet, a diet presently recommended to IBS sufferers. That being said, the reason we take all fruit out, as compared to the FODMAP diet, is that we also want to cut the supply of all sugar to the conbiotics™ (bad bugs) that are residing in the D-Spot. Cut the food supply and they will die and leave the system. Daily practice of castor oil packs are also very helpful when we're trying to get rid of conbiotics™, because castor oil has been shown to break down biofilm[297] [298] [299], a sticky protective layer that conbiotics™ can create to stop us from killing them. Very few natural substances have the ability to break it down, but no surprise - castor oil is one of them!

Fruits you will miss during the Clean phase:

- Banana

- Apples

- Pineapple

- Berries

- Cherries

- Pears

etc.

The ones I like and don't restrict on the Clean phase are the following. **Enjoy as much as you like!**

- Coconut

- Lemon and Lime

- Avocado

Why?

Coconut is a fruit that is chock full of good, healthy saturated fats. Contrary to popular belief, saturated fats are good for you when they come from a vegetable source, as opposed to animal sources. We need these fats as we clean house. Coconut oil is a natural anti-microbial, anti-yeast and specifically helps to treat Candida albicans, the notorious D-Spot damager[300].

Coconut oil seems to help improve lipid profile, increasing good cholesterol (HDL) and reducing waist circumference in patients with coronary artery disease[301]. It has the potential to improve memory, prevent and manage Alzheimers disease[302] and because it's a fat, it keeps us satiated while fasting more so than other oils, but less than medium chain triglycerides alone[303].

Avocado is a fruit very close to my heart. I aim to eat it as often as possible. It is composed mainly of soluble fiber and fat. The type of soluble fiber found in avocado is one that is excellent for improving overall health. The official serving of avocado is 1/5 of the fruit or rather 30g; most people consume one half which is 68 grams. Its claim to fame is that it improves absorbability of lipid based nutrients, improves maternal milk and health, helps with weight management and overall improvement in longevity. It's a superfood second to none[304] [305].

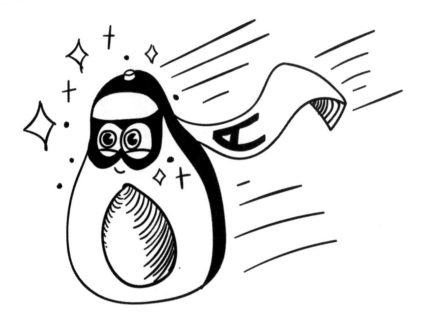

I'm sure you've heard of the saying when life gives you lemons, make lemonade! Besides lemonade, there are so many ways that lemons and limes contribute to living well. This is why these fruits made it into the D-Spot Meal Practice. Many people think that these fruits naturally cleanse your body because of their vitamin C content, antioxidants and citrus flavonoids[306] that support weight loss and reduction of inflammation. But in fact, they do so many more amazing things in the body, most of which directly affect your D-Spot!

Lemon and lime have a component known as D-limonene which has been shown to be effective at improving our D-Spot by reducing gastric acid, improving conditions such as gastroesophageal reflux disease

(GERD)[307], as well as optimizing peristalsis and normalizing D-Spot transit time[308].

Citrus fruits, in general, have an inhibitory action on **pancreatic lipase.** Other known pancreatic lipase inhibitors include green tea and rice bran[309] [310]. Inhibition of the digestive enzyme lipase which breaks down fat is presently being studied as one of the ways that citrus fruits aid in weight loss and obesity management[311] [312].

During the Clean phase we use lemon and lime as a substitute for vinegar in our salad dressings. Remember to put a little extra healthy oil than you normally do if you use lemon or lime, because you want to make sure you get enough of the healthy fats absorbed.

Use the whole fruit and nothing but the fruit! Peels of lemon and lime are great sources of the minerals calcium and magnesium[313]. Modified citrus pectin, which comes from the peel and pulp of citrus fruits, has been shown to be very helpful for people dealing with cancer. From helping to reduce the risk of metastasis to improving chemotherapeutic side effects, they seem to have benefits across multiple forms of human cancers[314].

One very interesting piece of research which I stumbled upon, was that a specific type of lime, the kaffir lime, inhibits streptoccoccus biofilm formation. This is huge as biofilm is what makes bacteria, viruses and yeast stick to our bodies and tissues[315]. As mentioned before, castor oil packs are an amazing tool to help reduce biofilm, one of the reasons why I love them so much and they are the ancestral key to our health. Make sure you are practicing them nightly!

How do you get the maximum benefit out of your lemonade? It seems that hot water extraction of phenolic compounds from citrus fruits is as effective as methanol extraction[316]. So the next time you boil some hot water or tea, don't forget to drop in some lemon or lime!

Dairy

We are the only mammal that drinks another mammal's milk. Odd, right? Milk is the product of conception and is meant to be the food of life for the baby of the species. Why then, do we insist on breastfeeding from the cow? It's just not natural and the reactivity we are experiencing as a whole to the milk, especially in children, speaks for itself[317].

Dairy from cows is thick and mucus forming. Comparing it to polyphenols found in green tea which greatly enhance the viscoelasticity of the mucus on the surface of the intestine[318], the opposite is true for dairy. It is acidic in nature, as it comes from an animal source, and it contains acidic amino acids. This can make it detrimental to your overall health.

Cow, goat and sheep dairy alternatives exist by the truckload these days and commercial trends have shown sales in the animal dairy industry declining, while sales in the plant-based dairy alternatives category are climbing[319].

There are some relevant health reasons to give up the dairy. In Germany, cancer patients are recommended to stop consuming dairy, since dairy is made to grow things, and the last thing that you want is to promote growth in the bodies of cancer patients. You can get calcium from many other foods. The research at this point is unclear whether there is a positive or negative association with dairy consumption and cancer risk, but some research indicates that it may be inversely related[320].

Some plant-based dairy alternatives are:

- Almond milk

- Rice milk

- Oat milk

- Quinoa milk

- Cashew milk

- Hemp milk

- Coconut milk

These days, there exists so many options that it's just a matter of choosing which is of your liking, and which does not fall into your food sensitivities category. Many people are allergic or sensitive to almond, so be careful of this choice. My favourite due to low allergenicity is coconut, plus, the taste is great.

One thing to be cautious about is the ingredient carageenan. Most proactive dairy alternative companies have already removed this thickening agent from their products. The reason is that there is conflict as to whether there are benefits of carageenan, or if it is just an inert filler[321] that may actually have negative effects on health[322] such as gastrointestinal upset, inflammation and possible links to cancer. So, at this point, since there is so much discrepancy, better to be safe than sorry. If possible, avoidance of this ingredient in foods is probably your best bet.

Avoid these proteins!

By far, pork, processed meats, and tuna are the protein sources that are least recommended to consume, each for their own very distinct reasons.

Pork and processed meats are often put under the umbrella of red meat. It seems consumption of pork and processed meat (most made from pork), increases cancer risk[323]. Out of all red meats, processed meats seem to confer the greatest risk[324]. It conveys a high risk that is associated to cancers of the esophagus[325].

Pork also happens to be so closely related to human tissue, which is one of the reasons that pork insulin is most often used for diabetic patients[326]. Pork is closely related to human tissue, and it is proposed to be difficult to digest. On ingesting pork, there is potential that our body actually recognizes it as its own tissues, and for certain sensitive people this can result in an autoimmune response - a fancy word for the body attacking itself.

In general, people who have an autoimmune condition like rheumatoid arthritis, multiple sclerosis, Crohn's disease and other conditions, tend to react with an increasing intensity of their condition to many foods, including pork[327]. One school of thought says that allergenic proteins, such as pork, tend to take longer to digest[328]. Those foods should be avoided. Personally, I feel that pork, even if you do not have an autoimmune condition, is a very reactive food and should be avoided, and consumed only infrequently. If only, because it takes longer to digest and acts like a big heavy weight in our bellies.

In certain religious faiths such as Judaism and Islam, pork is strictly avoided[329]. It is considered a dirty food, and in fact this is supported by multiple cases of transmission of diseases via the consumption of pork such as Hepatitis E[330], toxoplasmosis, dysentery, and amebiasis[331]. Pork seems to be a vector of disease transmission and a meat best avoided.

Tuna, on the other hand, is disliked because of its contamination with heavy metals, specifically mercury. Because tuna is such a large, fatty fish, and the ocean is seriously polluted with heavy metals, the amount of time that tuna is exposed and absorbing these heavy metals makes it a cess pool of mercury. Apparently, even more important than the amount of time in water for the degree of contamination is actually the location from which the fish was found[332]. Remember, toxins are stored in fat! Oh, Sh*t!

Packaging makes a difference too. The greatest levels of mercury are found within the fresh fish. When it is canned and olive oil is added, it contains the most amount of mercury, and when pickled, the least. Could this be the reason why we tend to have more 'pickling' and fermentation occurring in our bodies when we are loaded with heavy metals? Could this be a self-protecting mechanism? The jury is still out but we do know that canned tuna in water is found to be somewhere in the middle for levels of mercury[333].

Mercury is a very harmful substance that is neurotoxic and damages our nervous system. In addition, it negatively impacts our immune system and hormonal balance. Pregnant women are recommended to stay away from fish in general to avoid it causing harm to their babies whose nervous systems are in development. If it has that impact on babies, what then do you think it does to us?

What are our options?

Best Protein Choices

Not all protein is created equally. In fact, each protein source is very unique in the time it takes to digest, the amount of protein you get per gram, the vitamins or minerals obtained for the D-Spot and its allergic potential. All protein has a very unique imprint.

The most important factor in protein is its ability to digest quickly. From a scientific perspective, digestion is not 100% well understood. When it comes to digestion and our D-Spot, a lot still remains unknown, like the mystery of the black hole. What we know comes from experience and trial and error, both personally and with patients.

Animal protein, in general, takes longer to break down than vegetarian versions when they are in their natural form. When these proteins are broken down into powders, both the animal and plant source become equal in digestibility.

Many proteins, especially those that are animal sourced seem to confer a good amount of essential nutrients that are difficult to get from other food sources. They are an important source of vitamins and minerals such as B12 and zinc that are not necessarily found in high enough levels in foods other than animal protein[334].

The protein with the least potential for allergenicity and becoming more popular these days is wild game. So if you know people who hunt and are willing to share their loot... make sure to stay on their good side! Wild game has consumed food in its natural environment, not the preselected nutrition received by farmed and caged animals. This natural selection of food allows them to have an Omega fatty level that is extremely healthy. Their digestibility and nutrient profile is excellent, and their allergenicity is greatly reduced since we haven't had extreme exposure to these products. They may be fattier meats and many people say they have a 'gamey' taste but they are so good for you. So it's time to develop your wild taste buds!

Spice up your life

Food is better with flavour. This is not rocket science. But what can be a science on its own is flavouring your food to make simple meals extraordinary. Each herb and spice has unique therapeutic benefits. They contain pharmaconutrients that can enhance digestion, improve absorption and most importantly, make your food TASTE great!

My all time favourite is **pepper**!! Simple, plain old pepper! Don't be afraid of this spice and life-extending herb! Pepper contains piperine, the active component of the herb that improves absorption of nutrients in your food. That's right, adding pepper to a meal improves your bodily absorption of the nutrients. How's that for a spice that's got kick?

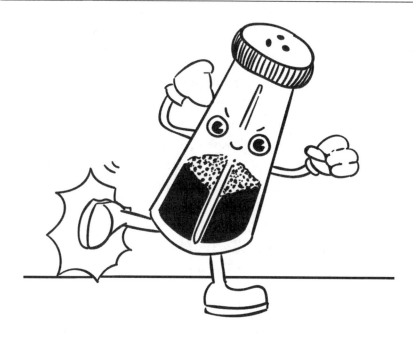

Here are a few of my favourite spices that not only add flavour but therapeutic value. These include:

Cumin: Many people say, "Everything tastes better with cumin"! I just throw it in as much food as possible. Cumin is a wonderful digestive aid.

Coriander: The dried and ground seed of the cilantro plant. Cilantro leaves are used therapeutically to help with detoxification. In animal studies, coriander has shown to be effective at protecting the liver and reducing lead concentration in poisoned rats as compared to a positive control group[335]. It is also a strong antioxidant and antimicrobial.

Pepper: I said it before and I'll say it again, pepper makes everything better! In fact, piperine helps you to better absorb all foodstuff and supplements[336]. Whenever you add pepper to a meal, it'll augment your absorption of the nutrients within the food. It is anti-inflammatory, immune-modulating, antioxidant, anti-carcinogenic, anti-ulcer and much more. It may surprisingly also be of benefit in drug absorption including antibiotics as well as chemotherapeutic agents and more[337].

This simple herb that hangs out at the kitchen table is a superhero in disguise.

Chocolate: Actually considered a phenolic rich food[338] that can be used as an herb. It is therapeutic in many ways and was used by the Aztec and Mayan cultures to adorn and as a spice for mole sauce over chicken, with paprika and hot peppers. Chocolate these days is used as a treat. Some chocolate has been manipulated into pure sugar and has none of the benefits of the real thing. So watch your source, and indulge in 100% cocoa. Some of the newest findings include the flavonoids of chocolate improving cognition[339], insulin sensitivity[340] and hormonal and immune balance. Chocolate has also shown to be helpful in improving heart function and lipid metabolism[341]. Can you believe it? Chocolate truly is the food of the gods[342].

Curcumin: (A.K.A. turmeric) is a Godsend. It has so many wonderful functions, such as improving glutathione levels in the body, enhancing liver detoxification and reducing inflammation. Just make sure to always combine it with some type of fat like coconut oil (because you'll likely be cooking!) and pepper. The fat and pepper help to enhance its absorption.

Wise words:

1. Watch when you cook with turmeric, as it will stain everything yellow including your nails, your countertops and anything that comes into contact with it!

2. Curcumin can affect the phases of liver detoxification. It may slow down phase 1 and phase 2 enzymes, and this is not good if you are sensitive to caffeine or have other low functioning enzymes due to genetics[343]. A build up of toxins can ensue.

3. Certain people have a food sensitivity to curcumin. I myself cannot tolerate it as it irritates my gut and this is something that I have noticed in practice time and again.

4. Curcumin needs to be cycled in and out of diet to prevent sensitivities to it.

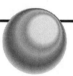

PEARL OF WISDOM

Make a half pepper half turmeric shaker for your dinner table. That way, it's easily accessible to add it to your food & you'll reap the benefits of curcumin!

Rosemary: A source of rosmarinic acid, a component that helps to reduce inflammation within the D-Spot[344]. Inflammation aggravates an unhealthy gut and contributes to its problems. In addition, it also contains carnosol, a component that augments your natural detox agent, good ole' glutathione[345], and is also an anti-cancer and anti-inflammatory agent[346]. Rosemary is a key ingredient in Eau de Throne™, the After You Poo Parfum™ because it heals the gut and has all these wonderful benefits. It smells divine, you always want to keep your bathroom stocked!

Garlic: A super herb/vegetable used to season most, if not all dishes. It is a gold mine of sulfur, a component of food that helps with detoxification and cleansing. Studies show that garlic helps to prevent glycation, which is when sugar causes damage to our cells[347]. Some people have problems digesting and utilizing foods high in sulfur because they are low in the mineral molybdenum. Molybdenum and sulfur work together[348]. Sulfur foods can also be a bit irritating for the D-Spot but are less problematic if cooked.

Onion: Another super herb/vegetable, onion is often paired with garlic to provide flavour to food. It is also high in sulfur and works to improve detoxification functions. When you're low in molybdenum, you will be unable to properly process sulfur[349]. Some people can tolerate cooked onions better than garlic because the heat deactivates the excess sulfur. These foods/spices are supportive in helping the body fight a variety of conditions[350].

Ginger: With so many amazing benefits it's hard to name them all! Ginger is anti-inflammatory, anti-cancer, a carminative (meaning that it helps to improve digestion), anti-nausea and so much more[351]. If you're the type that gets nausea with your green tea, perhaps taking a ginger supplement or adding ginger slices into your tea will help. On top of that there are multiple minute intercellular communication effects that ginger triggers, much like all the other herbs. It is also a warming herb that can help with building internal heat and health.

Cayenne Pepper: Once popularized by the Master Cleanse, this is a herb that enhances circulation as well as metabolism. But most importantly, cayenne pepper can increase your HCl. It improves digestive weakness[352] by bringing heat to the stomach, optimizing stomach acid. It mediates this by stimulating the vagus nerve whose job is to start up the entire digestive process[353]. It is also an anti-inflammatory and rubefacient analgesic, which means that it reduces pain by causing irritation. The mechanism of action is that the active ingredient in cayenne pepper, capsaicin, is a Substance P antagonist[354]. Substance P is a neuropeptide involved in the transmission of pain information. This is good stuff, start adding it to all of your meals!

Dill: One of my favourite carminatives! Dill has a wonderful taste that can be added raw to any salad or steamed vegetable dish. It helps you to digest your food, is anti-inflammatory, reduces flatulence, provides minerals and is a recognized antibacterial for the mouth and gut[355].

Cinnamon: A delicious herb that you can add to just about anything, especially to your smoothies. Its main claim to fame is its blood sugar regulating ability, which means it'll keep your insulin and blood sugar balanced as you heal your D-Spot. It also reduces colic, dyspepsia, and digestive weakness. It's anti-microbial, can reduce the filaments and plaques that cause Alzheimer's disease, protects the liver, and aids wound healing[356]. Add it to as many things as you can so that you can reap its far-reaching benefits!

Fluids For Your Healing

No clean health practice plan is complete without a discussion of the fluids you should be consuming during your D-Spot Meal Practice. Obviously, the rules continue to apply to avoid coffee, but what should we be drinking as we heal our D-Spots?

Certain teas have major health benefits. In my opinion, green tea is the best and second is red rooibos tea. We've spoken a lot about green tea already. It heals the gut, stimulates the liver cleansing function and a host of other amazing things.

There are other teas that are herbal and very beneficial as well. Here are a few of my favourite herbal teas:

Rooibos Tea: Red bush tea, otherwise known as rooibos tea is one of the most therapeutic teas after green tea. Rooibos tea is pronounced many different ways and I'm sure I have not yet mastered the true pronunciation. This tea is unique in that it is one of the only teas that increases the body's natural production of glutathione, a feat only achieved by a few other substances that we ingest.

Glutathione is the master detoxification agent and is best absorbed via a nutrient infusion. Certain supplements like NAC and magnesium help your body to be better at producing glutathione, but rooibos tea does it all on its own. It helps to reduce oxidative stress on the body[357] and it is also caffeine free! Yippee, so you can consume at any time of the day without worrying about caffeine that may keep you up at night or negatively affect detoxification of your liver. Drink this tea as often as you can as the health benefits are huge! Another way to preserve glutathione levels in the body is your daily castor oil pack practice, it is so important[358]!

Peppermint: Commonly used to help with soothing the D-Spot and digestion. It is to be avoided if you have reflux as mint will actually aggravate the situation. Otherwise, it is great as a digestive after meals and of course, as most herbs are, it is high in antioxidants. Research suggests that the availability of the essential oil of peppermint is best found in the tea as opposed to herbal supplementation[359].

Licorice: This is an adaptogenic and immune-modulatory herb which has shown to be beneficial in gastrointestinal disorders such as ulcerative colitis[360]. It helps your body adapt to stress and can help with regulation of the oh-so-important immune system within the D-Spot. It can be fairly stimulating, which makes this tea better if taken in the earlier part of the day. Licorice is also known as a natural antiviral[361]. It is especially beneficial if you are feeling low energy during the Clean phase, or if you feel you may be coming down with something.

Chamomile: This is the relaxant of all teas, the one that is in every mother and grandmother's cabinet. This tea is great for calming down your nerves. It has been studied in generalized anxiety disorders (GAD) and found to be beneficial[362]. Relaxing the nervous system allows the body to heal, while stress prevents healing. So the more you can tweak your health practice to reduce stress, the better your healing will be.

Nettle: This tea is a favourite among naturopaths. Why? Because nettle is chock full of so many benefits. It has a high mineral profile, nourishes the body, feeds the soul and cleanses the liver. It is caffeine free and one of the most traditional remedies known to man. Nettle is number one!

Caution:

1. The taste isn't fabulous but its benefits are so numerous, so who cares!

2. Since nettle is so good at absorbing minerals from its environment, it is also efficient at storing heavy metals too[363]. It is known to be one of the teas with the highest contaminant level, so you must absolutely know and trust your source on this one or it can be bad news. To remind you, heavy metals contribute to a higher level of bad bacteria and yeast overgrowth. Remember the tuna? When fermented, it has less metal contamination because fermentation is an organism's protective mechanism against metals.

Red raspberry tea: This tea is known as a woman's hormone regulator but is also very high in antioxidants[364]. It's been shown to have a protective effect on the digestive tract, helping to safeguard the cells of the throat and colon. It is said to also increase glutathione[365].

Hibiscus or sour tea: Commonly referred to as the heart healthy herb, hibiscus tea is bright red in color and helps to regulate heart beat and nourish the blood. It also seems to act as a pancreatic alpha-amylase and intestinal α-glucosidase inhibitor in the D-Spot[366]. That means that it reduces the amount of absorption of sugar into the blood. Although good for diabetics, it's not very good if you have a dysbiotic D-Spot because that leaves all the sugar in the gut, a recipe for disaster! It seems however, to be a good source of iron and copper[367] and increases total antioxidant capacity even greater than green tea[368]. So, all things considered, it would be a welcome addition to your tea cabinet.

Sarsasparilla: This tea is best known as the flavoring for root beer. Remember the old cowboy movies? When they sat at the bar, they asked for a, "Sarsasparilla, please?" Ironically, much like beer, sarsasparilla has estrogen and hormone regulating effects[369]. Men shouldn't have too much, as it could effect hormone balance. The thing with sarsasparilla is that it tastes so delicious that it's hard to say no, and with no caffeine or sugar, it's a great way to get your sweetness fix! It is now being researched for potential anti-cancer effects[370].

Carbonated Water: An awesome alternative to soft drinks if you want something that will tickle your throat. It shouldn't be over consumed, as the carbonation can be acidifying to our tissues, but used appropriately it is an excellent tool for a healthy lifestyle. When out with friends, I recommend to get it in a tumbler and it will look like you are having a drink. Add lemon and lime and a pinch of stevia and you have your own fun, non-alcoholic, refreshing beverage.

Water: Obviously the number one drink of choice during your Clean phase! Water is the universal solvent and as such, should be consumed frequently as the aim is to flush the system and remove all the impurities. I often get the question which water is best, reverse osmosis, distilled, Brita or home filtration systems. The reality is that our water truly needs to be purified from the fluoride that is added to it and the chlorine that is used to clean it. These are elements that don't belong in our body in excessive amounts. On top of these aspects, our water supply now contains an enormous amount of hormones. People who use birth control pills or other hormone medicine end up urinating it into our water supply. Unfortunately, this does not get filtered out with city water cleaning systems.

The gold standard to get your water clean and pure is reverse osmosis. This is a four star filtration system that has an impermeable membrane which does not allow any pollutant into the water, including pesticides and hormones. The biggest issue with reverse osmosis water is the fact that it can be a huge waste of water. Roughly four litres of water are wasted for every litre that is produced. However, it is the most effective way to remove harmful substances from water. Many people find reverse osmosis water tasteless, and this is true as all the minerals have been removed. This is not a bad thing, as we do not absorb the minerals in our water. We absorb minerals via our food such as fruits and vegetables that we consume, not through our water.

Supplement Clean Up

It's time to go through your cabinets and purge all the low quality supplements you may have, or the ones that don't serve you. Most people need to work on the basics and build the foundation before diving in to the big kahuna supplements. An example of this is taking an herb, but not seeing any of the beneficial effects because you may be deficient in vitamins and minerals that are needed to utilize said herb. You must have a good base of nutrients in the body in order for specialized supplementation to be effective.

Tuning up your supplementation regime is a vital aspect of your personal health practice and more important than you can imagine. Sometimes the best way to implement an effective supplement regime is to start from scratch. Many of our new patients want to finish the supplements they may already be taking. At times this is okay, as long as they are high quality supplements, delivering what they promise and taken at the right time. I have taken many supplements over the years, and some felt as if I would be better off taking nothing, because it felt like they did nothing. Now I notice when I stop my supplements for a few days, I can feel a shift in my body and I realize that I feel much better when I am consistent with taking them. Good quality supplements nourish, provide energy, support a healthy immune system and balance the brain, nerves and hormones. These are all keys to a great life.

One by one, I want you to become aware of what is in your supplements in order to embark on a fresh, new journey to health. You should be using only the highest quality supplements for your body, your temple! You were given only one, to dance, sing and live in - feed it the very best you can!

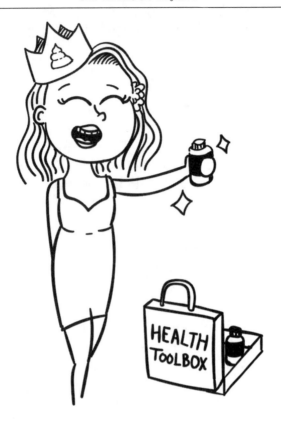

Here is the process of going from average supplementation to the best of the best.

Step 1: Supplements in tablet or chewable form

- Most of the time tablets and chewables are full of fillers. Also, most of us have such a weak digestive fire that we are not able to absorb much from this form of supplement.

- Fat soluble vitamins such as vitamin D should never be in tablet form. It must be suspended in a fat in order to be absorbed!

- Certain nutrients that need to be absorbed in the mouth, such as B12 and GABA, are the exceptions to this rule as the tablet form is conducive to absorption.

- Certain herbs are sometimes complexed in a tablet, this is not ideal but in some cases may be necessary.

Step 2: Supplements containing the following ingredients

- **Food coloring:** An ingredient that is artificial, unnecessary and concerning with regards to optimal health[371].

- **Cyanocobalamin:** A cheap form of vitamin B12, cyanocobalamin is usually a good indicator of poor quality of the supplement.

- **Fructooligosaccharides (FOS):** Added into probiotic formulas as a 'prebiotic' when in fact, they just irritate the gut lining and feed bad bacteria as well as the good. Avoid these in supplements, you get enough in your food!

Step 3: Supplements with the following ingredients have special considerations

- **Vitamin E:** A full spectrum of tocopherols with tocotrienols should be included to avoid depletion of any one of them, as supplementation with only a few can cause other forms to become depleted. Certain forms of vitamin E are protective against cancer and others are not[372].

- **Boulardii:** Saccromyces boulardii is the active form of this yeast, however, in certain supplements the cerevisiae form is used, which has no therapeutic benefit.

- **Folic Acid:** This is the form of vitamin B9 that accumulates in people who have a MTHFR genetic alteration and can be harmful. The best form to consume to prevent any issues is the

5MTHF or a natural folate that is sourced from vegetables like broccoli.

Always read the ingredients and if in doubt, ask a naturopathic doctor to assess the quality of a supplement before purchasing it.

The other conundrum when buying supplements is that they often have WAY too many ingredients in them. They may make many health claims on the label based on the choice of ingredients, but the ingredients are not in the correct therapeutic dosages to produce that effect. Therefore, they may not actually be doing you any good. A therapeutic dosage is the dosage at which an ingredient exerts an effect on the body. Taking very small amounts of herbs or nutrients may mildly support you but will not create significant changes.

Nutrients and supplements are medicine, just like food is medicine. It is important to take the right ones for your body in the right amount. I often find myself cutting my patients back from tons of vitamins and putting them on exactly the right ones for them. Remember though, to make great changes, it requires great effort and at times that correlates to taking more supplements than you are used to. Specific supplementation should only be for a limited period of time and then you wean from there.

Clean Supplements

During this phase, supplements gently begin to clean and tone the gut. In addition, supplements begin to encourage detoxification and energy so we can build the system up.

There are certain supplements that you can expect to be on for life. Some you may not start right away, but rather later. Timing is very important in protocols. Fish oils are an example. I rarely start my patients on these immediately (depending on the circumstance), but rather later on for maintenance and it becomes part of their life long supplement regime. What should be a base in your life practice are the following: Probiotics, digestive enzymes, multivitamin, multimineral, B complex, fish oils and an alkalinizing agent.

These supplements provide the basic building blocks for our bodies to maintain health. Our bodies are complex systems, and when you are trying to create change you need all the fundamental building blocks in place in order for the healing power of nature to do its job. You may think that's a lot of supplements to be taking, but remember these aren't drugs, they are health promoting nutrient powerhouses! With the rise of industry our food and soil has become so depleted that we simply do not get as much as we need from the foods we are eating, which makes supplementation essential for optimal health.

Remember, if you want drastic change it requires drastic effort. Supplements can provide the necessary support when they are of exceptional quality, in the proper amount, and at the right time. So during this phase that really resets your gut, increased supplementation and higher dosages are needed. You will stop certain ones after the Clean phase when you move into the Calm phase. You should already be taking a probiotic and an alkalinizing agent.

Probiotic

Probiotics help to keep the gut bugs in the right balance and spectrum. In order to begin the process of resetting the gut it's absolutely imperative to have a probiotic in your supplement regime. Often times people think that eating yogurt or kefir is enough, but if you remember from before, they may actually affect the gut negatively and won't help with repopulation!

The reason why probiotics should become a longterm supplement is because typically, we are not eating 100% organic, non-genetically-modified foods. GMO foods have typically been sprayed with glyphosate, a pesticide that causes damage to microbial communities, including the ones in your gut[373]. It weakens and damages your healthy gut bacteria[374]. When you eat genetically modified foods, this means that your good gut bugs are constantly being compromised.

Probiotics for healing the gut in a specific way need to contain certain strains in the right amounts. They also need to be dairy-free, or you negate the hard work that you are doing with the D-Spot Meal Practice.

Probiotics also need to contain Bifido bacteria in large strains, because this increases the amount of butyrate produced in the gut which supports increased natural inoculation of these strains of bacteria[375]. Bifido bacteria are a very important component of a healthy gut and research suggests that these strains of bacteria may have the most beneficial effect[376].

There is another amazing benefit of probiotics. When you have a healthy bacterial spectrum your body is less prone to absorbing the bad things like heavy metals and anti-nutrients such as cadmium[377]. Probiotics, no matter how you package it, help to protect and strengthen the gut.

This first prescription will help to start on stabilizing the gut microbiome. They are best taken on an empty stomach and in combination with an alkalinizing agent. You will likely already be on these two supplements since they were discussed in the Connect phase.

Alkalinizers

Alkalinization is incredibly important to the body because every area, including the D-Spot, has a highly regulated pH level. The body is a series of compartments that interconnect and work with each other to keep the balance. You should already be taking an alkalinizing agent as it was discussed in the Connect section.

The compartments start in the hollow tube of the D-Spot where gap junctions and the cell lining of the gut allow movement. Then you move into the extracellular space which contains a matrix of the connective tissue, the proteoglycans and hyaluronic acid. This serves as a molecular sieve that allows things to move. Finally, there is an intracellular space which is where all the magic happens in the body. Both nutrients and garbage travel on the two body super highways known as the lymphatic and circulatory systems.

The pH can push things in and out of the body. For example, an alkaline pH in the D-Spot will help the probiotics you are taking to propagate and stick in the D-Spot. Vitamin C further increases the improvement of gut health and may prevent growths in the colon and possibly prevention of cancer[378].

Alkalinization also has a multitude of other benefits including improving your overall health and reducing inflammation.

Zinc Carnosine and Demulcent

Part of healing the gut is to actually nourish the gastric lining. Zinc carnosine is incredibly important as it is required to heal a dysfunctional gut lining. It has been shown to enhance conventional treatments for digestive concerns significantly[379]. 25% of the population is deficient in zinc[380] so it is absolutely necessary to supplement to have a healthy gut lining.

Signs that you may be deficient or low include having blue eyes, a change in or lack of smell and taste and a great sensitivity to light. Zinc is used in the receptors of these nervous system functions, so when you are deficient, their functions decline.

Zinc supports the immune system as well as the mind, so there are many crossover benefits with zinc supplements. It is best if you can find a supplement that includes demulcents, which are herbs such as marshmallow that help soothe inflammation and make it easier for the ever important probiotics to make roots in the healthy gut lining. Zinc should always be taken with food otherwise it may cause nausea.

Antimicrobial

When you are resetting the gut bacteria, it's not sufficient to only add probiotics to the mix, you must also work on getting rid of bad microbes as well. Antimicrobials help to kill off bad bacteria and reset the environment of the gut.

Herbs such as berberine and black walnut help to kill off bacteria in the gut so that you can repopulate with the good bacteria in your probiotic formula. Berberine is a must-have in any antimicrobial formula for two reasons. First off, it improves the gut microbiota to the extent that it helps with treatment of diabetes[381]. Secondly, it has a protective effect on the D-Spot's mucosal membrane[382].

It takes time, skill and strategy to get it right. Your antimicrobials should be taken AWAY from your probiotics, always, otherwise they negate each other. The other thing is that you shouldn't be taking these all the time. Why would you? I've had many patients that I've had to counsel for being addicted to their grapefruit seed extract or oil of oregano that they swear by, every day. It simply doesn't make sense to constantly attack the bugs. Do it right, do it in cycle, and then let the body do the rest.

B Complex

The importance of B vitamins should not be underestimated. They are critical co-factors in the nervous system and the production of neurotransmitters (the things that make us feel happy or sad). They strengthen the adrenal, stress and immune response, they clear out toxins and hormones and give our bodies cellular energy. Most importantly, they help to heal the D-Spot lining. We couldn't live without these B-eautiful things!

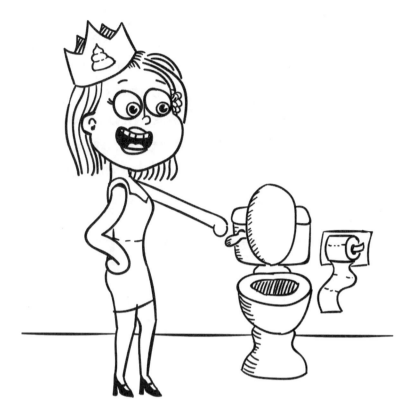

The more stressed you are the greater amount of B vitamins you require. They are water soluble so they will not become toxic to you. In clinic, we often give injections to patients of the B vitamins, because the levels required are so high that we can't always get it from oral supplementation. B12 is one of the big keys and many times we give extra B12 on top of a B complex, especially because it is one of the key B vitamins for D-Spot health.

> Never take a B vitamin on its own. You must always take a complex because you want to make sure you don't deplete any of the B vitamins. **Too much of one can lead to depletion of another.** They should work in concert with each other.

Multimineral Formula

Minerals are necessary to make the machine move. An exceptional multimineral is one that is iron-free and provides the minerals required to keep your body in balance. Minerals in both small and large quantities, depending on the mineral, are required to keep the detoxification and cleansing functions of the body working optimally.

We have to be careful of getting too much iron or copper. Many people, especially menopausal women or people taking certain medications, can develop health conditions from too much iron or excesses of copper.

An excess in iron is mainly hereditary and can cause an iron storage disease where it is stored in the vital organs of the body. Iron is a heavy metal that can damage the body. The other thing is that most people know if they are iron deficient or "anemic", because hopefully they have been assessed by their doctor if they have felt incredibly fatigued.

Iron, as a side note, also isn't recommended when you are trying to reset your gut bacteria. Iron feeds bacteria and yeast[383], so if you have an overgrowth, this could be one of the factors that is affecting you. You may also be anemic because your body is intelligently hiding the excess bacteria so you can survive.

An excess in copper is carcinogenic[384] and since many people live in old houses, they will have exposure to copper wiring. It is best to leave copper out of a mineral supplement so as to avoid an excess. At times it may be in very specific supplements only because those supplements require copper for activity.

Multivitamin

A multivitamin completes the spectrum of nutrients by supporting with sufficient amounts of trace vitamins and minerals so nothing is missing. We need all the nutrients, vitamins and minerals for our system since it is a unit. Unfortunately, the present state of our food is devitalized in nutrients so it can't serve us as it did previously. Plus, we are overwhelmed with too much stress, both emotional and physical.

Digestive Enzymes

Digestive enzymes are important as we age, because over time, we lose the ability to have excellent digestibility. For some, this comes earlier than others. Mainly, it is due to the fact that since we have weak digestion, we can't break down the protein necessary to absorb, in order to have the raw material needed to make the digestive enzymes! The weaker the D-Spot, the greater the need for digestive enzymes.

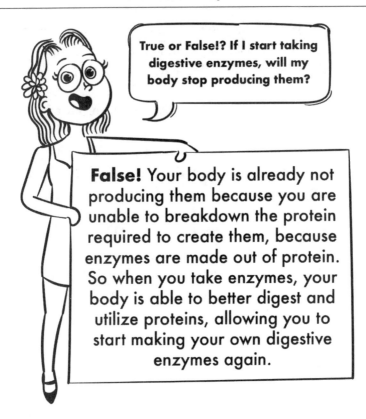

True or False!? If I start taking digestive enzymes, will my body stop producing them?

False! Your body is already not producing them because you are unable to breakdown the protein required to create them, because enzymes are made out of protein. So when you take enzymes, your body is able to better digest and utilize proteins, allowing you to start making your own digestive enzymes again.

Vitamin D

Sunshine, A.K.A. vitamin D, is essential for life! I mention it here because vitamin D deficiency is something I see all the time in clinical practice and it's an absolutely CRUCIAL nutrient for good health. The healthy level of vitamin D is between 160-220 nmol/L. It's typically safe to supplement with vitamin D, but an excess is possible (although rare), so it's always best to test first. Find out more about vitamin D in chapter 8!

So there you have it, you've successfully worked your way through the Clean, and now it's your time to move into the Calm.

Whatever time you commit to this Clean phase (start with two weeks then try to stretch it to four to six weeks!), know it is worth it, because you are SO worth it! Always remember to check in with your health care practitioner before undertaking new health strategies. This information is not meant to treat, cure or prevent any disease and is for educational purposes.

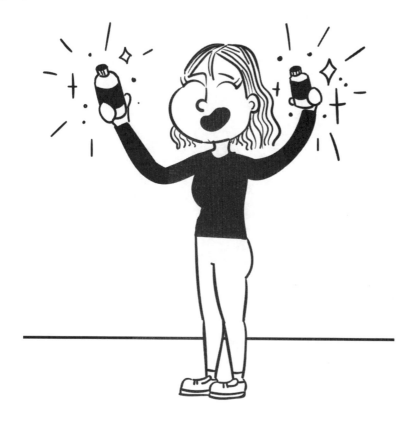

CHAPTER 8

CALM LIKE BUDDHA

When you think of calm, you might imagine Buddha, sitting cross-legged, a faint peaceful smile on his face, meditating. This phase is perhaps the most important, because a calm state is crucial for your body to heal.

Here you are, eating the most amazing diet ever and you've got the timing all right. Nothing passes your lips unless it's approved on the D-Spot Meal Practice. You've got this, or so you think. Why then do you, after a little time on this amazing practice, start to feel crappy again and why on earth would you buy a book that starts to make you feel crappy?

It's because there is an untold secret that no one has ever told you in any health book or any program (or at least from what I've read and experienced)...

I've seen countless patients go through this. They feel amazing for the first little while, and then the benefits of the first steps to changing their life seem to wear off. They don't actually wear off, but what happens, is your body becomes adjusted to this new state of health. This becomes your new normal, so the "dirt" that hasn't been cleaned up in your foundation from the beginning now starts to muddle things up and you feel, well, sh*tty.

It's like a relationship with a partner that doesn't feel right. You may try to pretend that everything is good, say the right things that you read in a book, do the loving actions like Oprah says to do and go through the motions. But the problems that got you into an energetic funk to begin with are still there, until you get the courage to talk about the issues and the sh*t that is unpleasant. It's the only way to fix things. You've got to clean up the dirt both emotionally and physically. Your D-Spot health is exactly like that.

With my IBS, it got really aggravated after a time when I was doing everything right. Aggravation also occurs when I'm not being conscious of the practices I will talk about in this chapter. I like to think, practice doesn't make perfect, practice makes progress.

My rhythm rocked, my exercise patterns were stable and my food choices were completely stellar. I had this down. I had the "connecting" and "cleaning" phases in the bag. There I was, the supposed picture of health, the preacher of healing. Suddenly, boom! I'm in the toilet more times than I care to count, and likely more than even most of my patients. If you remember from the beginning, my challenge has always been anxiety and stress getting the best of me, more so than I'd like to admit.

So needless to say, like every other human being out there, when sh*t hits the fan like this, it's really easy to get discouraged. This is exactly why I'm sharing this story with you, because it's just part of what often happens. If you go in with that expectation and are aware of it when it happens then you can react accordingly. My life was best summed up by my teenager's wise words, "How come mom is the healthiest of us all but seems to have the most problems going to the bathroom, not to mention leaving deliciously smelling gas gifts all over the home?".

Talk about discouraging, no? Don't get discouraged, because this is part and parcel of the entire process. Without this moment of setback, you can't evolve to where you need to be. For me, and many of my patients, we all think it's 100% about how we are eating and about the food. However, that my dear friends is just the tip of the iceberg. What really moves the needle is the work we all need to do to achieve the CALM.

Your D-Spot is now being fed the right foods at the right time. But the biggest and most crucial part is creating the space for it to be calm, free of debris and garbage, free of physical and proverbial irritation.

In order to do this, it will take all of the superhuman power that we all have inside, and we have to accept the struggle. We all love and admire superheroes, but why?

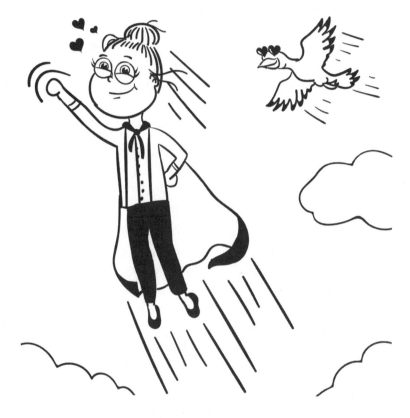

It's because they struggle through the worst of it, to come out victorious. You are exactly like that. Life is no cake walk, it's a journey through different versions of struggle. Some struggles are easier to deal with and others take all your efforts. The bottom line is you can overcome all struggles if you put your mind to it. It will take our dedication and determination to wanting to live a better life. We can all do it.

You're probably shaking in your chairs now, thinking this chapter is going to be true penance, the worst of the worst and the hardest to achieve. Fear not my friends; be bold! (I'm not a meanie anyway).

So, if the rhythms and diet are the easy part, what is the final stage? It was my missing link, I hadn't gotten down into the aspect of my self care that is number one, the most crucial, and number two, the hardest to keep on track because it takes motivation and a will to maintain the practices that will keep you balanced. But the REWARD is huge! Calmness brings us ultimate clarity! In fact, all three steps intertwined and combined are the foundations for clarity, in the things that we want for our life and the way we want to live.

In this final Calm phase, the focus shifts to the creation of physical and mental calmness. Many may think that this calm is achieved by going to a spa or hiding out in a desolate area away from all of civilization. Albeit, this is one way to achieve calm. But our biggest challenge is achieving calm amidst all of the chaos in our modern day lives. This translates into moving the baggage that is tripping us up and getting in the way of connecting our body, mind and soul.

The focus here is not so much on food, as in the previous chapters, but more about keeping our beautiful temples free of debris for life. Debris or garbage, can come in many unlikely shapes and forms, and to achieve calmness, both the mental and physical 'basura' needs to be moved out for health optimization.

Getting deep into your guts requires more than just a physical diet. Here is where you will learn to dominate your D-Spot and make it divine through minding your mind. We will refine your food, add in physical therapies and focus on the mental mindset which are the keys in this phase, as we really want to exert the healing power of nature.

When your D-Spot is calm, your focus and clarity on your health and your life is tremendous. Many of the practices to follow can be added into your plan at any time. However, many times and for many of us, we first must focus on the physical body before getting to this stage. It is much easier to do the physical work or labour before getting into these aspects of healing. You will find the health practices to follow start with the physical aspects and can be used long term or short term depending on you and your needs. These will help you in the acute situations of constipation or feeling "toxic", stressed, and therefore not calm. Cleaning the D-Spot is the first step to achieving calm. These practices can be used one at a time to build your health practice or in combination. Here you will need to listen to your body and figure out what is right for you. Just always keep an open mind. Some of these practices may scare you, but I promise, I wouldn't write about them, or be a "frequent flyer" if they weren't great for you.

Take my hand; let's do this, you superhuman, you! You're steps away from achieving and relishing in the fruits of all of your labour. You've got this, and I'm guiding you. One practice at a time. Stay CALM and carry on.

D-Spot Bowel Movement Magic

Movement is necessary for life and if things still aren't in royal flow like you'd like them to be, we begin to add in the tools to enhance how you go. This way we can regain our calm. How do we know that the baby we just birthed is alive? She or he cries. That cry is the creation of movement of air in and out of the lungs. A healthy D-Spot requires movement like all other parts of the body. It's such an important part that it needs to be the first thing you do to help reset the D-Spot in the Calm phase. Movement for the D-Spot is sometimes described as clearing the bowels or cleansing.

When you think of the word cleansing many people picture sitting on the throne, flushing all your brown royal gems away. The reality is that the bowel movement function and the elimination of waste is cleansing, but it's a completely natural function and one we can't live without!

Green Tea: Components of green tea have a laxative effect. Pu'er tea, a form of green tea, contains strictinin which has shown effectiveness as a laxative by stimulating an increase in transit time in the small intestine[385]. Other studies have shown an increase in hormones like motilin, gastrin and acetylcholine enzyme[386], which stimulate the bowel. If you focus on the fasting period to increase the amount and varieties of green tea, plus the fluid you are drinking, this will help enormously to get things moving and grooving in your D-Spot.

Why do you think I got you started on the green tea in the Connect phase? I find this can work stronger than a laxative at times, especially if you drink enough tea and if you don't halt the process by eating. Every time you eat, you halt the major motility complex, MMC, which is the in-between eating, movement maker of the D-Spot. Food signals it to stop dead in its tracks and causes the food in your intestine to sit and fester. This is so that you don't poop your pants when having dinner. The signal for it to begin again is the emptying of the stomach contents into the small intestine[387]. So imagine the impact of fasting with green tea that stimulates both the hormones and your natural digestive reflexes. You basically have a recipe for bowel movement bonanza!

Bowel movements are of the utmost importance for your longterm health practice. Especially when you are working to tune up your D-Spot. If you are not going daily, ideally 1-3 times per day or a large stool that spans from your elbow to your wrist, your elimination is not effective. As mentioned above, things begin to fester in the deep dark recesses of the intestine and your body's response to it is simply to keep your metabolism and digestive byproducts in your D-Spot, where these toxic elements recirculate back into the body. It's an incredible ecosystem after all, and always in search of balance. The only problem with this is that it increases the overload on your system. This is called endotoxicity. Basically, what's inside of you is creating toxicity.

Maintaining your health is about making sure that the bowels are moving, that your D-Spot has a dynamic ebb and flow. This is the whole reason behind this book, your first step to health, and my other books to follow (The Movement Meditation, Eat Sleep Poop, etc...) will address deeper problems, but the intent of this book is to be the first gateway to help people heal. It's exactly what I do in my practice with patients. To take charge of one of their most basic functions and change how their health is evolving. I'm talking to you, yes you. You are in charge and you can change the evolution of your health and how your D-Spot is cleansing!

Some people find themselves on a tight schedule with their bowels. They go every morning after that "delish" little morning coffee. So what happens if we remove the coffee from your present practice? You may stop going, but to prevent that, make sure to stock up on your green tea or warm water. Warm water works as well as coffee to stimulate rectal tone[388]. Others are in the boat where they never go to the bathroom, they may make a trip every three to four days. So the key is to either start the flow or prepare yourself in case your flow falls off. All the tips in this chapter will really help you to gain your balance and calm in the D-Spot.

Castor Oil Packs

Castor oil packs work to relax the system, allowing you to have a better flowing bowel movement. You may be seeing a trend at this point, that relaxation of the bowel improves elimination from the D-Spot. Your deductions are correct, Sherlock! Whatever you can do to reduce the stress on the D-Spot will help you to get good flow. Enter my all time favourite old school naturopathic tool, the legendary castor oil pack. It was originally popularized by famed intuitive bedside healer Edgar Cayce, but its history dates back to Ancient Egypt, Asia and Greece, where even Hippocrates, the father of medicine, worked with them.

I owe castor oil packs my life. At the end of my third year of naturopathic school, I got dreadfully ill. Probably from a combination of too much stress, too much studying and too much political school dogma, along with too little creativity. Creativity is what keeps the fire alive in my heart and in yours too. I was forced to bed rest and faced to delay a semester of my internship. I was completely devastated.

I remember having just finished up my semester and participating in a class that taught treatment protocols for all conditions, called Naturopathic Foundations. There was one treatment that stood out as it was applied across the board, for all conditions, and that was the castor oil pack.

The problem was that they were messy and no one would comply with the treatments. So many naturopaths would opt to not recommend this incredibly valuable treatment, or they would opt for the lazy person's version, which instead of using a compress to do the castor oil packs, they would just rub the oil onto their skin (which I learned years later took away some of the very important aspects of the treatment).

To calm myself, as I was on bed rest healing, I started to sew. My first attempt was to make a tool to make the castor oil packs easy and clean to do. After all, I had started doing them every night, going to bed with them, and I didn't want to make a mess.

SO… as necessity is the mother of all invention, I invented a pack. And with the help of my business partner/engineer/boyfriend, we brought this newly designed pack to market. It is still one of my pride and joys and something that I birthed into this world. Fast forward to years later. We had broken up and I found there were things that needed tweaking on the pack. So I went back to the drawing board and fixed all of the problems with the old pack and my new Queen of the Thrones™ pack was born!

This inexpensive, quirky and simple treatment has such profound effects. It's hard to believe at times. I have seen patients on their death bed get relief from applying this pack on the abdomen. My goal is for us to never lose this treatment, because fancy, new, shiny things are always appearing, but they rarely work like the tried, tested and true legendary therapies.

So how should it be used? This grass roots topical treatment should be adopted as a regular health practice because it helps return the body to balance by enhancing its natural rhythm, coordinating the body's regulatory systems and connecting you to your source. Plus, there are real physical benefits for those of us who suffer from digestive issues and here they are:

Constipation, Bloating, Diarrhea and Irritable Bowel: We should "move" everyday. If we go too much or too little, and are really uncomfortable or feel pregnant even though we are not, there are troubles down under! When you have a bowel movement you should feel as though you have completely evacuated what's inside of you, and if you don't, you may be constipated. Castor oil packs help with that[389]. They also reduce the bloating and sensation of an irritated bowel. What if you are the other extreme? They help with that too. If you go too much they help to slow down the transit time by relaxing your gut[390].

Biofilm Breakdown: One of castor oil's main modes of action is to break down biofilm. Biofilm is a protective layer that bacteria creates so that it cannot be killed. Studies testing castor oil in comparison to conventional denture cleaners demonstrate that this mystical oil works better in the body to break down the layer of biofilm that protects the bad bugs (A.K.A. conbiotics™)[391 392 393]. This helps you to reset your D-Spot bacteria and reduce your bloat! All in all, this health practice is worth its weight in gold, I can't emphasize that enough.

Liver Cleanse: When your liver is working overtime, which is likely the case for all of us in this day and age; metabolism, digestion, elimination and hormones can all be thrown out of balance. These days we can't run, and we certainly can't hide as there are toxins everywhere we go. In the food we eat, the air we breathe, the products we put on our bodies and everything else that we do. Our best superhero weapon is to consistently adopt health practices that cleanse our bodies. The castor oil pack is one of those tools. Castor oil has been shown to help preserve our body's glutathione levels[394]. Glutathione is our master detoxifying agent that helps move waste products out of our bodies like heavy metals and toxins. For some people, increased levels of toxicity show up as high cholesterol. Castor oil packs have been shown to help with reduction of cholesterol[395]. Doing a castor oil pack regularly will keep toxins moving out of our system.

Core Inflammation Control: If you're gaining weight in your belly, you feel like you are busting out or you're consistently feeling back pain, then you likely have swelling in your gut and core. Regular use of a castor oil pack will help to reduce the inflammation[396] and stress that is causing swelling in your body. This will also help to improve immune system function with use[397]. Place it over the swollen area or on the liver to help quell this inflammation and regulate your immune system. It is very helpful to use castor oil packs over swollen joints as well.

Period and Hormonal Problems: If your periods are heavy, you feel the bloat and cramps til' the cows come home and may also be acting like a wee bit of a royal bitch, you likely have premenstrual syndrome (PMS). Castor oil packs will help your period along. They help your tissues relax, therefore improving the whole hormonal experience for you and those around you. They are safe to use during menstruation and some practitioners don't recommend during pregnancy, but I do. However, it's only because I know my patients' health histories and many of them have been doing the packs for eons and I can monitor them. So if you're new to castor oil packs, pregnancy may not be the time to start something new.

Hormonal problems such as ovarian cysts, uterine fibroids and cystic breasts have all been treated and responded well to castor oil packs.

Relaxation and Resilience: Castor oil packs are like the escape button on your computer. They quickly switch you into the relaxed state to encourage rest[398] and sleep which is where healing occurs[399]. Having periods of stress and then relax are important for us to be resilient. The more you practise relaxation, the better you are at achieving it in a moment's notice when sh*t hits the fan. Castor oil packs also help to naturally stimulate dopamine[400], our "feel good" neurotransmitter, and oxytocin[401], our love and attachment hormone. So pretty, pretty please practise your castor oil packs, you are royally worth it!

There are so many benefits of castor oil packs that absolutely everyone should be incorporating them into their daily health practice! The issue with the traditional way of doing castor oil packs is how time consuming and messy they are. This is why I created the Queen of the Thrones™ castor oil pack and here is why it is the absolute best tool for this practice:

Just so you can press the easy button. Easier than ever before, this innovation is a heat-less, less-mess, 3-step treatment pack that I designed to increase compliance and keep life easy. It's as easy as **1-2-3, C-O-P!** (**C**astor **O**il **P**ack)

No chemicals, no way. Re-designed to make a once messy treatment cleaner, it's also clean for your body. Designed with luxurious organic cotton flannel to gently caress your skin, and a protective outer layer of polyurethane (PUL). This PUL is made without any chemicals and is eco and health friendly.

You're curvy, your pack should be too. Because you aren't square or triangle, your pack shouldn't be either. It is designed to fit your curves, the way that it should.

One size fits all. Your liver is the size of a football. Your pack should be larger than that area to cover multiple organs and get the most benefit out of the treatment.

Visit www.drmarisol.com to get your Queen Kit today that includes the castor oil pack!

Look, if you can't get your hands on the organic **Queen of the Thrones™ castor oil pack** that will make your life super easy, then these are the instructions for one to be done with a simple flannel.

1. Make sure to use only **organic, chemical-free cotton** (organic means free of pesticides, not free of chemicals; always ask the manufacturer to ensure the material has not been chemically treated with flame retardants).

2. Warm the cotton flannel in a double boiler, with a hot water bottle, or on the heating vent (this is optional).

3. Add 2-4 tbsp of **100% pure, certified organic, cold-pressed, hexane-free, extra virgin castor oil** that is stored in a dark **GLASS** bottle at room temperature.

4. Place cotton flannel on body part requiring treatment (ie. over liver, abdomen, bowels, pelvic area, joint, etc.).

5. Lie down and relax for one hour or overnight.

6. Remove and store in a glass container in the fridge. Repeat for next treatment.

Note: ALWAYS buy your castor oil 100% pure, organic, cold-pressed, hexane-free and bottled in GLASS. Castor oil is an excellent carrier oil and can absorb toxins from being bottled in plastic and from poor farming and manufacturing processes. **We definitely don't want to be absorbing these toxins into our bodies!**

Essential Oils

Essential oils can be helpful for healing the gut as well. Eau de Throne™ the After You Poo Parfum™ is created with organic essential oils of lavender, rosemary, clove and limonene. These oils disinfect the air and also have incredible healing qualities.

- **Lavender:** Anti-septic, anti-inflammatory, anti-viral, calming, sleep-inducing

- **Rosemary:** Anti-septic, anti-inflammatory, promotes healthy estrogen metabolism, antioxidant, improves circulation, aids digestion, anti-cramping

- **Clove:** Anti-septic, improves digestion, reduces gas & bloating, anti-fungal, strong antioxidant

- **Limonene:** Terpene from lemon peel - excellent for GERD, aids digestion.

Not only does Eau de Throne™ support digestion and calm the nervous system, it's also an 'adult potty training tool' because since it is sprayed after you poo, it trains you to get in the habit of looking at your stools and analyzing them. Get to know those Legends in your Throne!

Movement for Movement

Movement is life. Without movement, we rapidly shrivel up and die. When we move we bring life to all areas of our bodies. We flow with blood, oxygen and nutrients and we let go of all the metabolic byproducts that each of our millions of cells produce. Flow in and out brings us life. Create the flow in your life.

Because we are living in a sedentary society, most of us sit on our butts all day long and simply do not move. Without physical movement of our limbs, our body has a difficult time creating physiological movement of all types, including bowel movements.

Movement is a physiological need just as much as breathing. When you have movement, there is life. The only time there is no movement is within death.

Having the discipline to create regular scheduled movement in your life is of the utmost importance. Think small things first. Park farther away so that you can walk a bit further at the grocery store. Take the flight of stairs instead of the elevator. While you blow dry your hair, try squatting, whatever! Hey, why not even just start to dance when no one is watching, if you prefer?

Infuse movement into your life as a discipline and it will soon become a major indulgence for you. Focus on the consistency of creating a disciplined routine and commit to it. That's all it takes and you will be surprised what a few moments a day can produce in the long run. Your D-Spot will thank you for it.

Back to Basics - Breath Will Move Your Bowels!

Move with breath. Most people breathe up into their chests instead of deeply into their bellies. The big issue with this is that if you are not breathing deeply into your belly, you're not utilizing your diaphragm to massage your D-Spot organs. This massaging action from the diaphragm actually helps to get the bowels moving. The human body is just incredible. All needs to be in tune, especially with the diaphragm as it connects all the internal organs[402].

Every action of the body has multiple synergistic effects. As an example, the other major benefit of beginning to take deep belly breaths is that it relaxes our nervous system. It moves your body and takes it from the stressed state of the sympathetic into the relaxed parasympathetic. This relaxed nervous system state is where the D-Spot moves. The parasympathetic nervous system connections go straight to the gut and command it to cleanse via peristalsis movements (the ebb and flow contractions of the D-Spot).

Three of my favourite beginner breathing exercises are deep diaphragmatic breathing, square boxed breathing and alternate nostril breathing. They are easy to do, can be done anywhere, and with practice, can help you to easily flow into breathing deeply on a regular basis, even when you are stressed. In general, they are a great tool to reduce stress in your life.

Deep diaphragmatic breathing is all about getting to know your breath in the relaxed state. How you breathe in the relaxed state is very different from how you breathe in the stressed state. Stressed state breathing is up into your chest, relaxed state breathing is deep into your belly and expands your chest into your diaphragm and pushes down into your D-Spot. The best way to get a feel for this type of breathing is to attempt it lying down.

Steps to Deep Diaphragmatic Breathing:

1. Lie down on your back.

2. Place your hand on your belly.

3. Take a deep breath in from your NOSE, and feel it push your hand up into the air as your belly expands.

4. Exhale slowly through your NOSE and feel your hand fall deep into your D-Spot.

5. Repeat, focusing on elongating the inhale and the exhale.

6. Repeat 10-20 times.

Practise this as often as possible. Ideally, I would recommend to do it ten to twenty times in the morning and repeat again before you go to bed at night. It's like anything, the more that you practice this technique the easier it will be for your body to fall into it and repeat it naturally throughout the day. With all tools in health we want to make it a practice, so that eventually, it is super natural and so are you!

Boxed Breathing

The evolution of boxed breathing just takes your deep diaphragmatic breathing to the next level by adding imagery and counting. This easy breathing technique elongates the breath and helps you to learn to focus on deep diaphragmatic breaths that move the D-Spot and help you to retain more oxygen from each breath that you take. Therefore, you are actually getting increasing nutrition in the form of oxygenation from every breath you take. Oxygen is an ultimate nutrient. You cannot live without it and you require it to rock your world and give you the inspiration you need to live a full life.

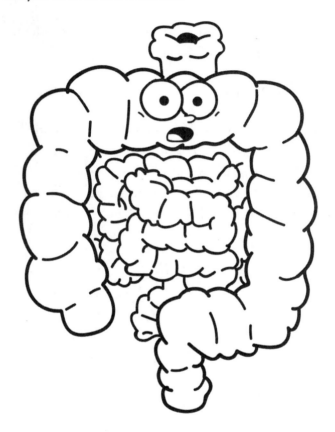

Steps to Boxed Breathing:

1. Picture a box in your head. Coincidentally, it is similar to what your large intestine looks like.

2. With four counts, inhale deeply into your lungs and draw the line in your mind from south to north (like the ascending colon in the image above).

3. Then from west to east for four counts, hold your breath (transverse colon at the top of image from left to right)

4. Now from north to south for four counts to exhale (descending colon on the right of image)

5. Then from east to west, hold your breath (sigmoid, rectum and anus, at the bottom of image)

6. Repeat 10-20 times.

If you have issues with picturing the box (intestine) initially you can draw it on a piece of paper to look at it, while you practise. Eventually it'll be burned into your brain and you will just be able to think of it. Picturing the intestine really helps to nourish the area because you will be sending really great vibes directly to where you need it most!

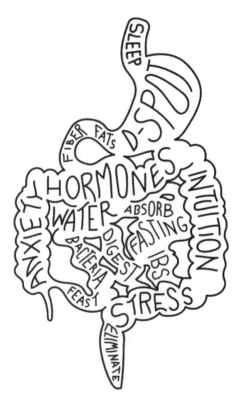

Alternate Nostril Breathing

An easy technique but one that you have to pay attention to, is alternate nostril breathing[403].

It begins with the warm up circulation breath. Inhale through the right nostril, holding your breath and then exhale through the mouth. You are to feel strength coming into your body and the life force from the air. Make sure to block your left nostril with your left hand. Repeat this three times all through the right nostril. This breath breathes energy into your body and it circulates the air.

It is followed by the alternate nostril breathing, inhaling via the left nostril, holding the breath, then exhaling via the right nostril and holding your breath, each time blocking the alternate nostril. You will feel these breaths enlighten your mind. These breaths are a lighter type breath. Repeat this three times, starting with the left nostril, the right nostril, and then the left again.

Breath is the inspiration of life. With each breath, always try to imagine yourself breathing in all the energy, goodness and beauty that the world and life have to offer. Take it all in because it is yours to enjoy!

Whichever breath practice you choose, repeat it frequently. Practise, practise, practise, because this is a health tool that you do not want to be without.

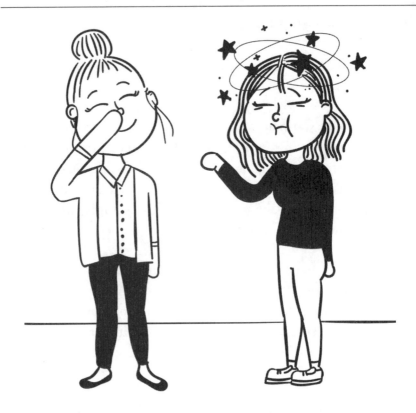

The Crowning of Your Royal Jewels!

Another issue is how we are sitting on the throne to have a movement. The modern day toilet isn't designed for an optimal poop.

Back in the paleolithic days, what did we do as a race? Easy! We squatted and then popped and moved on. As Mother Nature recommends, the easiest way for the crowning of our royal jewels to happen is to squat. This is known as the Paleo chair. The toilet only half squats us, if you put your bum on the seat. The other more ergonomic option is to stand on the toilet seat and squat and then you have the perfect position. But it's dangerous and not recommended, so don't do that!

Ironically, research presently doesn't suggest that squatting reduces your risk of colorectal cancer as opposed to regular toilet seats[404]. So why do it? As simple as this, it just makes sense to improve the mechanical way you go potty. The research may catch up to our squatting years later, and the solution is so easy. Just grab a small block or a stool and place it at your feet when you are owning your throne. I also like to use my 'poo pumps', my highest high heel shoes that put me at the perfect angle. A huge stack of books works too. Keep it in your bathroom and use it every time. Getting into this position opens up the lower sphincter which will make way for your poo! Hooray for savvy ergonomic stool hygiene!

Fiber

Many people ask me why I rarely speak about fiber when concerning the D-Spot, and simply the reason is this. If you're eating the way you've been instructed in the D-Spot Meal Practice in the Clean phase, you will be consuming plenty of fiber in a day, more so than you probably have had in your entire life.

When you cut out all the grains and you load up on fresh and cooked vegetables, you get a lot of roughage to help your body clear. That being said, there is a small minority of you that could use a little added encouragement in this department so it's important to note this here.

The recommended amount of dietary fiber is approximately 14g/1000kcal, so in a 2000 kcal diet, approximately 28g would be the ideal amount of daily fiber[405]. Would you believe that less than 3% of North Americans are achieving the daily recommended amount of fiber[406]? Unbelievable! So clearly, change in diet is first and paramount. When the diet is changed, you may like to add in a bit of extra roughage so you don't feel like being a cow and grazing all day. You can add in a good quality fiber supplement too, but real food is always best!

Please do try to stay away from certain fiber supplements, some of the most prescribed and advertised ones contain ingredients such as food colorings. These are irritants to the D-Spot, and although they may provide some roughage, they also come bearing bad gifts that leave the spot in disarray. *Oh, Sh*t!* Read your labels carefully.

Some people just want to keep their fiber simple and prefer to go with psyllium husk, which is another of my favourites. The great thing with adding fiber into the diet is that it significantly helps with fecal fat excretion[407]. This is a fancy term for fat coming out in your sh*t, and it's one of the ways that the body cleanses and also one of the reasons why I recommend to load up on good fats in the D-Spot Meal Practice. Fats move out the chemicals and bad stuff in our bodies. If we are deficient in fiber, then the fat simply recirculates. This would cause stress on our systems and would take us out of the Calm that we are trying to achieve

Water

I'm really hoping at this point, that water is the unwritten rule to getting healthy, and you are applying this practice daily. But if not, it definitely deserves mention. Your D-Spot thrives on water. It requires plenty of water for it to be healthy and have good flow.

If you don't drink water, don't expect your D-Spot to be happy. An arid desert there does nothing for your movement and it shouldn't ever resemble Arizona. You need to think of your D-Spot like the Florida everglades. You want it to be adequately hydrated and humid. If not, it simply won't function like it is meant to.

Keep in mind the dehydrating effects of black tea, coffee, sugary beverages and green tea (to a smaller extent). What I do to prevent the dehydration that can come with green tea, is that for each cup of green tea I consume, I drink the exact same amount of water. That keeps me guaranteed to flow!

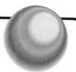

PEARL OF WISDOM

Pour half a cup of green tea & then fill the rest with water. This guarantees that you'll always have enough hydration!

Reverse osmosis is always your best choice. Be wary of well water because even if you have had it tested and it's not bad for you, they haven't tested all of the contaminants, and there could be junk in it that would not do your body good.

How much should you be drinking? You should be drinking at bare minimum, approximately 25ml/kg of body weight. This translates for a person who weighs 60kg or 136.4 lbs into approximately 1500ml of water in a day, or one and a half litres of water. If you're active, or live in the desert or a very dry home, you clearly need to increase this amount accordingly. Remember, this is the bare minimum!

Did you know that the study of water intake known as hydration is an entire area of nutritional research? Clearly, it's an important factor to our overall health and when it comes to our D-Spots we simply can't deny its importance[408]. Wash up your insides with water and don't you forget it. Drink as much as you can and always carry a few bottles with you so that you can hydrate at a moment's notice.

Supplemental ways to MOVE your D-Spot

When you've tried the breathing, the positioning and all the other steps above and still have no success, it's time to bring in the supplements to support your success.

These are two of my favourite tools that you can use, if being backed up is getting the better of you. Remember, fundamentally, there are more issues than simply efficiency, but this is a great way to get the ball rolling, so to say.

Magnesium, it only works if you take it!

Magnesium is required in many functions of the human body. There are more demands for this mineral than most others. When you're low on magnesium, your stool comes out in balls. Stress can deplete your magnesium levels, and let's face it, who doesn't have stress? In addition, certain classes of drugs notoriously deplete your levels of magnesium such as proton pump inhibitors which are used as antacids[409].

People taking these drugs have been known to have serious laboratory deficiencies of this vital nutrient. When it shows up in your labs, then you have a serious case of deficiency because most people may not be deficient in their lab values yet have a deficiency. This is because lab values, in general, don't necessarily show the true story when it comes to magnesium.

From women to men this deficiency is rampant, although more for women because of our hormonal surges and changes which require that we use up more magnesium. Boy, can we be complicated! Women are just more complicated you see, because of the orchestra of awesomeness (guys you're awesome too, just different) that we have going on that lets us bear children. I'm sure you would agree. Bottom line, magnesium is necessary no matter if you are male or female.

Now really, how does magnesium help your D-Spot?

Magnesium helps your D-Spot relax and move. How does it do it? It's an osmotic laxative that pulls fluid and water into the intestines. The fluid and water fills the colon and hydrates the stools, preparing them for evacuation. The dosage of magnesium required is extremely individualized and from day to day can change. This is because first with magnesium you will replete your deficiencies. Once repleted, you will hit the sweet spot that pushes you over the edge where magnesium is used as an osmotic laxative.

Magnesium is by far (along with castor oil packs, probiotics and green tea) one of the prescriptions I recommend the most. It's involved in over 300 enzymatic reactions in your body on top of its bowel moving osmotic function. With a daily dose of magnesium, your body is sure to calm down. And with it, your switch from the sympathetic stressed state to the parasympathetic rest and digest state is another way magnesium helps your D-Spot. It simply helps you to calm down.

I bet with magnesium, we have barely scratched the surface on all of its functions in the body. We don't know the half of them.

I often get the question, because there are so many forms of magnesium, which one is right for me? Which form of magnesium usually depends on you and your presenting symptoms and concerns.

Magnesium glycinate - this is one of my favourites for bowel health because it does triple duty. It works as an osmotic laxative. The glycine helps with phase two of liver detoxification and the function known as amino acid conjugation[410]. Glycine is also a powerful molecule that can calm the nervous system. Plus, this form of magnesium provides less bowel discomfort than magnesium citrate.

Magnesium malate is a form of magnesium that helps with pain sensations all over the body. It is frequently used for fibromyalgia and muscle pain. Malates are intermediates in the citric acid cycle, the energy production cycle of the body. Malic acid comes from apple or sour tasting tart fruits. It is used in the cosmetic industry[411] and in terms of natural health, thought to help the body to eliminate aluminum, a detrimental metal whose claim to fame is causing Alzheimer's plaques in the brain.

Magnesium threonate is used mainly for calming the mind and helping the brain. It is one of the newest forms of magnesium. It easily crosses the blood brain barrier and rapidly places you in an extremely relaxed state. Research demonstrates its ability to help with short term memory deficits associated with pain[412]. I enjoy this magnesium every night before going to bed after a busy night of work.

Magnesium citrate is commonly found in many mineral formulas. Citrates are very good at removing dietary oxalates for people who have a tendency to create kidney stones[413]. Citrates are also very good for detoxification. I personally find that citrate formulas can cause more bowel gas, and sometimes can be a bit uncomfortable when used to help your D-Spot move.

Magnesium carbonate is typically used in alkalization formulas and with vitamin C to alkalinize the acidity of the supplement. Because it reduces acidity so much in tissues, this translates into healthy bones in the body[414].

Milk of magnesia, otherwise known as magnesium hydroxide, is typically prescribed by a pharmacist to help the bowels move[415] and as an antacid. I've personally never prescribed this form of magnesium in my practice.

The winners are:

- For moving the bowels, both magnesium glycinate and magnesium malate

- For relaxation, magnesium threonate

- For alkalinizing, magnesium carbonate

- For detox and cleansing, magnesium citrate

So now that we know about the forms of magnesium, how do you go about challenging your bowels with magnesium?

Royal Magnesium Flush

You will need magnesium capsules or powder.

1. Before bed, take the lowest recommended dose of capsule or powder.

2. If no bowel movement the next day or if not loose, increase by one capsule or respective powder dose.

3. Continue increasing every night until you have loose bowels the next day.

4. If bowels become too loose, reduce by one capsule or by the respective amount of powder.

5. Maintain dose of magnesium in order to keep your bowels moving daily.

6. Augment as necessary if you notice you are not going. It could be a sign that you require more magnesium at that point due to an increase in hormones or exposure to toxins.

Vitamin C Lavage

The other supplement besides magnesium that can be used to stimulate your poo production is vitamin C. Some people prefer working with vitamin C in lieu of magnesium, it just depends on what works best for you.

Personally, I prefer magnesium over vitamin C as I find that the vitamin C lavage can cause some discomfort due to gas and irritation. Best to try out both and see which one works better for you.

Vitamin C offers its benefits in that it is one of our master antioxidants. Not only does vitamin C help with recycling the ever important master detox agent glutathione, but it protects our blood vessels, helps with the creation of collagen to keep us young and improves our immune system when we are sick.

Oral consumption of vitamin C, however, has its limits as it has an osmotic laxative effect after a certain dose. What's the dose? It's unknown, and just like magnesium, it is completely individual to each person. If you're sick and fighting something off, you would require much higher amounts than usual. Some people say it's above 10000 mg, but remember, it's individual so you have to figure out your sweet spot.

Vitamin C is an osmotic laxative at high doses which means that it pulls water into the body. Some people take such a high dose orally and get no benefit from it. This typically means that they are so deficient in vitamin C that their bodies are simply soaking it up in order to replenish the deficiency. Your body is extremely intuitive and knows what it needs and when it feels it, it soaks in.

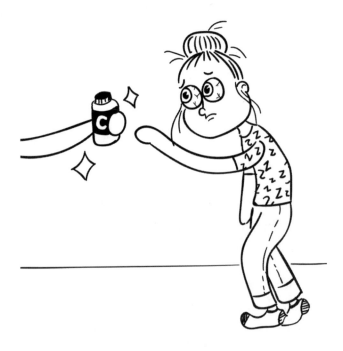

To do this, you will need vitamin C capsules or powder.

Typically, it is started with the lowest recommended dosage, one capsule or the respective amount of powder. If no movement happens, then it's titrated upwards (meaning a slowly increased dose), same as magnesium.

Please note that some people will experience gas, bloating and odd sensations in their bowels. This is normal as vitamin C pulls the water from other parts of the body to create the laxation.

The other thing is that if you have a fever or flu, or if you are sick, expect that you are going to need a lot more vitamin C than normal to make your bowels move.

Meditation

In chapter 5, we got into a deep discussion about how digestion is truly about how you are digesting your life. The D-Spot, as divine as it is, can be a source of much struggle for us, mainly because it is our centre of intuition. For some people, simply quieting their lifestyle by connecting with the tools from Chapter 6 and/or improving their digestion as in the Clean chapter is sufficient. For others, myself included, you need a couple of four by fours smacked straight onto your head for your D-Spot to get the picture and be sitting pretty.

When you haven't honed in on how to connect with your intuition, you end up leading a life full of anxiety, addiction and strife. One of the best ways to hone into your intuition and to let go of the addiction anxiety infinity loop is to adopt a meditation practice. For so many of us, it seems like an impossibility. Every time I ask a patient if they have tried it they all typically reply, "There is no way I can sit and not think, no way."

I believed this too. I used to think meditation was for weirdos, sitting on a cliff, drinking their green tea, or hippies who had nothing better to do.

Why on earth would I sit and be quiet? There is so much to do right here and right now. Even famous people like Arianne Huffington struggle with this thought. She is well known for her meditation prowess. There was a time when she didn't want to add another technique into her life but then realized that you don't do meditation, it does you.

For me, you could say that I was so busy with stuff, that I was doing a form of active presence meditation, one known as being mindful, "be here now". Although beneficial, it is not the same as actual meditation, and I'd say I was likely missing the mark as I was just too busy, with my mind being everywhere at once.

I remember the first time I tried meditation, back in naturopathic school. Again, it was because I had fallen dreadfully ill, and I was willing to do anything to get better. I remembered sitting in the middle of my condo, cross-legged, lights off, ready to do this thing. However, for a 'doer' like me, it's hard to sit there and 'doer nothing'.

I would get restless, trying to take deep breaths that I am sure were making me hyperventilate. With each breath I would get these weird tingly sensations in the lower part of my ribcage. It turned out I was never breathing deeply, so the tingling was all just oxygen going to places it hadn't been in a while. My mind was going everywhere, "What was that assignment I had to turn in?", "I can't believe she said that to me", "Shut-up! You're supposed to be quiet! Okay, refocus, take a deep breath". The inner chatter in my mind was giving me a headache and I definitely wasn't feeling zen.

But I persisted, and as we all know, persistence pays off. I also started doing meditation while wearing my castor oil pack. It was an enormous help to get me into the relaxed state.

Those tingles passed, the anxiety and nervousness subsided, and suddenly as I kept refocusing on my breath, all was feeling better. My thoughts quieted down, the tingles disappeared and I was feeling good.

I no longer felt like I was hyperventilating. When I finally opened my eyes, that felt like they were closed forever (it was actually only ten minutes), a new feeling flushed through my body. Well, not totally new, but a new high, a quiet, natural high flushed my system. I couldn't believe it. All was well with me and the world and all was great and grand. This was what zen felt like. Oh Sh*t!

It was the first time where I actually held a true state of quiet meditation and received the full effects. It was by far not my first try. All the other times I tried didn't end up that way, mostly because I got scared with all the new sensations, the tingling, and what felt like hyperventilation and the tightness in my pain points and chest. This, be forewarned, is completely normal, and I promise you it will pass. Keep on sticking with it and you will get through it. Hmm, sounds like a life proverb when so many realizations come to you while meditating. Don't do what I initially did, which was quite the opposite by giving up and then ending up frustrated, swearing that meditation was only for people in robes who are bald or have braids!

I'm not the only one who has adopted this practice and found that everything they wanted to manifest in their lives literally started to happen when they began to practice regularly. It really is that powerful. But there is the story of the Buddha, who was a sheltered, rich prince, then became a peasant. He lived both extremes, and within those extremes, realized that there was more to life.

That more to life was the quiet union of the body, mind and soul, along with the collective soul of the world, the connection to all that delivers more peace, happiness, prosperity and love than anything on this earth. That includes things like money, which many people feel is their *raison d'être*.

The understanding of the collective conscious and tuning in to your connection to the universe will profoundly change who you are. For some, it's their connection with God, Buddha, whatever they believe.

For others it's the universe. When you're connected, you become completely intuitive to your purpose, your path and your service to the greater good. The small stuff isn't important anymore and doesn't cause you stress. Why? Because you're on a mission.

On mission there is a balance between effort and ease. Why? Because things really aren't a struggle. They are in one sense, but because it's a struggle with purpose, it doesn't feel quite as tough. With no purpose, many of us are living on a merry-go-round of effort. Every little thing feels like you're climbing Mount Everest in the Himalayas, and it feels like you'll never get to the top.

My friends, you won't, and thank God, because you're not going in the right direction. Quieting your mind allows your temple to clean the mud and makes it that much easier to connect.

Cleanliness is next to Godliness. Amen!

There are many others who lived this way besides the Buddha. Edgar Cayce, a famed bedside healer actually used meditation as his life mission to help heal other people. He would intuit their treatment protocols. He also intuited the castor oil pack. He was said to be the founder of natural medicine and it all came from quieting his mind and connecting to the source. To find out more, see the Association for Research and Enlightenment in Virginia Beach. This is where I certified in meditation training. It's an incredible example of healing from an energetic perspective.

Oprah Winfrey, who has become an enlightened leader of our time stated, "From the stillness you can create your best work and your best life." You could say that she is an example of this. I forecast this woman becoming the first black female president, in my perfect world.

Another infamous genius, Jerry Seinfeld, who is well known for his unique dry sense of humour admits, "If you meditate you can get so much more work done." Who would think that this high stress New Yorker would be so sweet on meditation?

Then there is Katy Perry, mogul musician managing a team of 127, who writes all of her own amazingly creative music. She spoke of meditation, "For creative types, the only time your mind gets calm."

Madonna, who lives and breathes meditation in all its aspects, holds a regular practice and attributes a huge part of her success to meditation. She said, "Meditation showed me how much energy silence has."

Steve Jobs, the genius behind Apple, was a well known meditator as well. The list just goes on and on.

These stellar people all have something about them that makes you want to watch them, be around them, and stay on top of their every word. They are being themselves completely and bringing their best into this world. They are on a path on their journey. These people all demonstrate ultimate creativity. They are also the types that tend to suffer from an irritated bowel or gut problems if they are not tuned in. They likely found this out early on in their lives and adopted this wonderful tool into their practice as they found that it fed their creativity, calmed their anxiety and tuned them into their intuition.

If I could eventually quiet my mind, there is hope for all of you out there. All it takes is determination and practice and these are the first steps that I developed to help my patients adopt a practice.

1. Put on your Queen of the Thrones™ castor oil pack to relax and prepare your body.

2. Find a quiet space. At first you really need this, because all the sounds and interruptions will likely get the better of you. I see it every time I teach patients meditation. They are like dogs that see or hear "squirrel!" As you learn, making your environment hospitable and conducive will make it easier. As you progress, you will notice you will become skilled at blocking out all of the noise, even on a busy city bus.

3. Start with Tibetan bowls or chimes. These help to set the stage, again preparing you for success. The sound itself is very transportive and calming and said to help with connecting you to your source.

4. State your intention to those around you. Ask your family to leave you alone while you are in meditation.

5. Start with 10 minutes. Set a timer on your phone. It'll be the best way to get into the practice.

6. Let your mind think. WHAT!!?!? How can this be? Aren't you supposed to shut it all down? You can turn off the mind as much as you can stop the heart from beating or the blood from flowing in your veins. If you find any thought that ends up

going too deeply down the proverbial rabbit hole, you're making a mountain out of a molehill and this distracts from your goal.

7. When this happens, bring your focus back to your breath. Inhale and exhale. If at any moment you get distracted, remind yourself to go back to your breath. This will keep you grounded and in a good spot.

8. Keep on practicing - if at first you don't succeed, try and try again. Repeat daily, as often as possible.

9. Be open to what comes.

10. Get ready for a breakthrough.

This is a very basic meditation for you to get your feet wet. When you try this, remember to stay open to what comes. You can do this. Just commit and be consistent. BE STICKY!!

I encourage you to go deeper and check out another book of mine, The Movement Meditation. This delves into meditation and why it's so important, and has my technique known as the Infinity Flow Meditation which can take you into the deep dive of meditation much faster.

At the end of the day, there are things to which we must adapt. Then I learned the most important principle of my life which tied all of my work together. Cleanliness is next to Godliness, and then it all clicked.

Supplements for the Calm Phase

Since the focus shifts to keeping things calm, the supplements during this phase are focused on how to balance that by supporting the calm environment that you are creating.

It's important to continue the other supplements mentioned in previous chapters, as they are building a solid foundation. These final elements are the *pièce de résistance.* Eventually you will not be on all of these supplements, but initially it is very important, especially if you aren't getting results with diet alone.

The supplements to continue include:

A probiotic, alkalinizing agent, vitamin E, green tea with ECGC, B complex, multivitamin and multimineral, digestive enzyme and any of the more specific supplements pertaining to your unique body in the Connect and Clean phases. Antimicrobials should not be taken all the time.

Sometimes, in order to help with consistent reduction of stress levels and the ability to be more resilient, there are certain herbs and formulations known as adaptogens or adrenal formulas that can make a big difference in how your body responds to stress. The adrenal glands are the managers of your stress levels, but in severe, long term stressful situations they can hit their breaking point and get burned out. When this occurs, your other systems, like the D-Spot, will take over the burden. So, supporting the adrenals helps to maintain the calm we are trying to achieve. We discussed these in the Connect phase, but it is worthwhile to repeat them, as things may have changed in terms of how you are feeling, and perhaps you need to adjust which ones you are taking.

Adrenal Formulas

A common misconception is that all adrenal formulas are created equally and can be taken at any time of the day. We know differently, and armed with that knowledge we dose our adrenal formulas at different times of the day because of how they affect the natural sleep wake cycle, that is awakened with cortisol in the a.m. and put to bed by melatonin. We spoke about these formulas in the Connect phase of this book and as you have learned before, neurotransmitters, such as melatonin, play an intricate role in maintaining a healthy, optimal D-Spot.

Fish Oil

Fish oils can now be introduced, because there may already be an improvement in how your gut is feeling. They help with calming inflammation, as do most healthy oils. Fish oils have been well researched to demonstrate this.

Vitamin D-Vine

I'm saving the best for last here. We all know that Vitamin D is essential to life. The only thing is, until you begin to do a bit of work on your gut, vitamin D can sometimes be difficult to digest. It's worth it to start, however, because it is essential to so many balances in the body bank account.

Known as the sunshine vitamin, it helps us to absorb calcium[416] so we have strong bones. It also impacts our immune system health. As an example, an interesting study suggested that the ability to fight off infections such as Tuberculosis is dependent on vitamin D levels[417]. We know that sub-optimal levels of this powerful vitamin are found in inflammatory bowel disease[418] and food allergy[419].

Without vitamin D we experience hormone dysregulation, like thyroid[420] hormones, our blood pressure is higher[421] and we experience more anxiety, burnout[422] and depression. Studies also demonstrated that vitamin D levels are essential to prevent breast and colon cancer.

It's called the sunshine vitamin because we get it from the sun. But for some reason, no matter how much exposure we get, we may not be absorbing vitamin D or retaining optimum levels. Could pervasive wifi in our society be a contributor? Could high exposure to electrosmog be depleting our vitamin D levels[423]? Or the fact that in areas with higher pollution, vitamin D levels have been found to be lower in people[424].

The jury is still out and I'm sure there are multiple factors.

In our clinic, we have tracked and followed patients over the years with their vitamin D levels and to our surprise, so many are deficient and many times, worse over the summer months. Some patients wear sunscreen and others do not. However, the results seem to be the same. The only way to know is to get yourself tested. You should know your levels!

The healthy level of vitamin D is between 160-220 nmol/L.

An excess in vitamin D, although very rare, can happen, especially in patients that are supplementing. We always test first if giving a high dose. Otherwise, we err on the side of caution and give a low dose like 4-5 drops, or 4000-5000 IU daily, which seems to be a safe dose for most. But even still, you need to be careful. I have definitely experienced patients taking a low amount and having elevated levels of vitamin D, which is toxic. Please make sure you are testing with your healthcare provider before taking any doses of vitamin D.

The Most Important Calm Practices

An attitude of gratitude works miracles in your life. One of the easiest and most important practices that helps to heal your D-Spot and improve your life in general is a daily gratitude practice. I use my Grateful Dung™ Bracelet that is included in the Queen Kit before every meal to implement the Daily Dung Dining Practice, as follows:

1. Before meals, hold onto the black obsidian Swarovski crystal dung beetle bead

2. Name three things you are grateful for

3. Repeat this at every meal, expressing new things each time

This simple practice helps to move the body into the rest and digest state, ready to absorb the nourishment of your meal to come.

Chew Your Food!

Another awesome way to use the Grateful Dung™ Bracelet is to remind yourself to thoroughly chew your food. As mentioned earlier, digestion begins in the mouth and the more we chew our food, the easier it is for our stomachs to digest it. I touch each bead for every time I chew, going around the bracelet until I get back to where I started. This ensures that I'm chewing enough for awesome digestion!

Beauty Sleep

We already discussed the importance of getting good quality sleep but it's worth mentioning again because it is absolutely crucial to achieving Calm in your life. Make sure you have an awesome night time ritual to set yourself up for success. The Queen Kit includes the Beauty Sleep Eye Kit with an organic cotton eye mask, Cosmetic Castor Oil and a double ended applicator brush, to nourish the delicate skin around your eyes and promote natural melatonin production. I can't stress enough how powerful getting good sleep is!

Moving out of the Calm

So now, with all these lotions and potions and your commitment and consistency over the past weeks/months to staying connected, being clean, and calming your system, I can almost guarantee that you must be feeling quite well (as long as you put in the time and effort)!

Now what do we do to maintain this momentum? Do we have to live within such tight parameters for our whole life? Or can we get back to basics and keep it simple?

Now we move on into the Clarity phase, which is the result of the Connect, Clean and Calm phases. This will tie everything together and show you what your future looks like.

Onward and upward. When you take action, things just happen.

As always my friend, please consult your health care provider before beginning new health practices. This information is not meant to treat, cure or prevent disease and is for educational purposes.

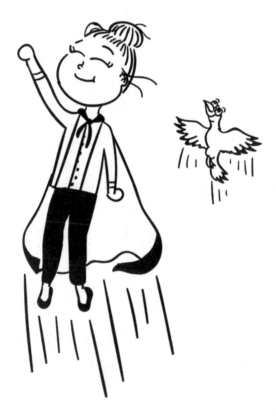

CHAPTER 9

THE CLARITY

You have done such amazing work. You should feel so proud. No doubt by now, you have had improvement. Sometimes, you may not even notice it because the changes can be so subtle over time and your new 'normal', feels, well exactly, normal! It's not until you get off practice for a period of time that you then experience the pain again.

Let's do a quick review of the steps you took:

You **Connected** like a Cavewoman, to your exercise, sleep and feeding habits and refined your new rhythms to be in balance.

You **Cleaned** like a Queen, by working at reducing the load on your D-Spot through the food that you eat and taking the appropriate supplements.

You **Calmed** like Buddha with castor oil packs, meditation and the right support for your stressed systems.

When you Connect, Clean, and Calm, you get Clarity. Now, how do you keep that Clarity? Do you need to maintain this plan for life?

You have worked so hard and fundamentally changed your system. What it takes to get better, it truly does take to stay better. You can definitely go off plan and make modifications so that it isn't as complex, but many of the basic principles I would encourage you to continue.

I get it. Life is tough. It's difficult to do all the things that you have to do, and to maintain a lifestyle like this takes work. But let me ask you.

Doesn't your unbalanced, unhealthy lifestyle also cause you work and drain your time?

Is it worth it to focus on maximizing your health and staying on plan? I think so. What's the price tag on your health? To feel good. Be full of energy. Be really, really alive! To me, it's priceless and worth the time and effort. Taking care of yourself helps you to be the best version of yourself, so you can show up for the people in your life who you care about. To truly illustrate the difference of committing the time and effort and maintaining the plan, let me look into my crystal ball and show you the future.

There are two avenues you can take.

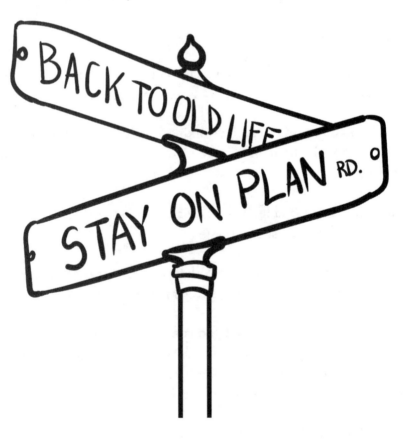

You can make the commitment to stay on plan, to adopt this as your lifestyle and your way of being. After all, isn't it amazing to have clarity? This is what life should be like.

Or you can decide to go back to your old life, into your old routines that aren't necessarily easier, but you're just more used to them. Wouldn't you agree? The thing is, you will eventually see the return of all of your symptoms and the return of your continued suffering. Why? Because a wine glass that you keep on filling with wine will eventually overflow, unless you pour it out or drink it! Your bad habits will begin to accumulate again and cause you to overflow with symptoms.

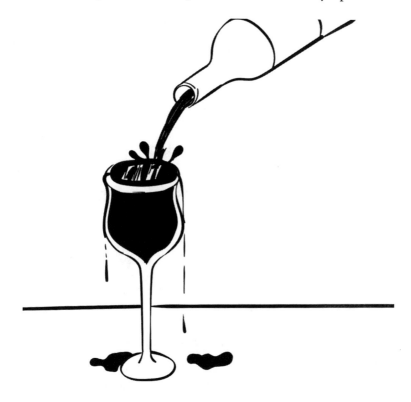

So my dear friends, the choice is yours. Do you want a life of clarity or a life of crap? I'm gonna bet you choose the first option. Good, stick to it. Don't lose your resolve.

When people, patients and friends go through the process of working to restore their D-Spot, they may think it'll be easier to go back to their old routines but honestly, it won't. You want to know why? It's because this has become your new habit. It takes merely a month to create a habit. Checkmark, you did that!

When you do introduce foods that you haven't eaten for a while or old sub-par life practices that you have worked to remove, they aren't going to feel too natural. But trust me and be careful. It's a slippery slope. Those are old habits, the neuronal networks for these habits still exist in your brain. So too much practicing and they will become natural again.

So the principle here is indulge, but always keep your discipline and introduce things just a little at a time. Please don't do what I initially did. After my first cleanse, the day I finished it, I basically binged! From drinking too much alcohol to drowning my face with sugar. How did I feel? I felt like sh*t, truly. So I decided to get right back on the cleanse.

Try to maintain the Connect, Clean and Calm principles throughout your lifetime. This information has given you Clarity. When you have Clarity, you can do better. If things aren't clear, you can't find your course, nor can you course-correct.

Let's get really clear on your steps moving forward.

D-Spot Maintenance

Fasting: This needs to be maintained as a practice, not every day, but regularly. Maybe you can consider doing it during the week and on the weekends take a break. But remember, fasting is a practice that keeps your body cleansing, and in our modern day world this is extremely important because we are overexposed to all types of toxins.

Exercise: There is no way around this one, you need to exercise regularly. Our bodies are made to move and this my dear friend is common sense but not common practice. Find one type of exercise that suits you. As mentioned before, just do a little each day. Sweat and get your heart rate up.

Sleep: Sleep resets our bodies and prepares us to be our best selves each and every day. It's mandatory to keep it well by maintaining your circadian rhythm and reducing your stress. How you do this depends on you. You now have plenty of tools, from supplements like adaptogens, to exercise and timing of your meals. I encourage you to create a nightly routine that works for you with castor oil packs, an eye mask, meditation, etc. You are prepared to make your sleep superb, or as I like to say, be sovereign over your sleep. Make sure to use your Queen of the Thrones™ Beauty Sleep Eye Kit every night to naturally produce melatonin but to also keep you looking like the beautiful cave women you are!

Diet: You are what you eat. So with that, obviously you are aware that the diet recommendations you have taken over the past bit with this book have brought you to have a different respect for what is healthy. Maintain the D-Spot Meal Practice as much as possible. However, you can introduce from time to time, starchy vegetables, grains, legumes, fruit, sugar and sweets. Just promise me, to not go hog wild. If you overdo it, like anything, what will happen is that little by little you will overwhelm your system. Eat lots of green leafy vegetables, hearty protein, and healthy fats. When you do introduce fruits, please be aware to not combine them with protein. So make sure that your fruit is on its own as the perfect snack. Look to the diet recommendations in the Connect phase, because this was your starting point and it is great for maintenance as well. Also don't forget the importance of simply CHEWING your food and using a gratitude practice before your meals. Use the Grateful Dung™ Bracelet as your guide.

Here's a note on food sensitivities. If you really want to reset them, especially those that are exposure sensitivities and not true sensitivities (true sensitivities will never change) it will take you at least one year of removing them from your diet. Not exclusively, but really focus on reduction for at least 1-3 months and then consuming for at least one year, only every 4-6 days. Of course, if you're practicing your castor oil packs and improving your body's natural relaxed state, you will speed up all of these healing processes. Still, to be on the safe side, I would recommend you take your time with this. Check out the resource page at the back of the book to find out more and get your testing.

Supplements: You will need to stay on supplements for life. That is the reality, since we don't get enough nutrients from our food. They help us to maintain a balanced state.

1. Probiotic

2. Alkalinizing agent

3. B Complex

4. Multimineral

5. Daily greens formula

6. Multivitamin

7. Fish oil

8. Vitamin D

9. Digestive enzymes

10. Vitamin E

11. Green tea

12. Castor oil packs (not a supplement but very important to improve absorption of all of the supplements you take!)

Practices for your Parasympathetic

Castor oil packs are the queen for your gut. They help to restore FAITH in our body's ability to heal, by supporting the five key foundations of health:

F - Function of digestion, absorption and elimination

A - Antioxidant status

I - Inflammation regulation

T - Tension and stress

H - Host microbial balance

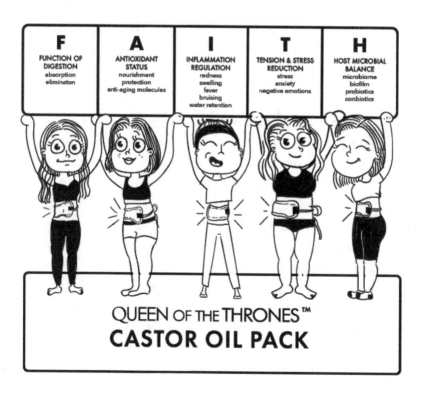

Deep breathing, gratitude practices with your Grateful Dung™ Bracelet, calming essential oils like in Eau de Throne™ and meditation will be mainstays no matter what, ingrained into the very fabric of your life. You're required to maintain these for your ongoing health.

Stress will knock you off your rocker every time. What I notice most with patients is when the stress hits, they need to focus even more on keeping their practices consistent. Because when you falter, that is when it becomes a slippery sliding slope back down into irritable bowel land.

Your D-Spot deserves your attention, and there is an important principle to observe here. What it took you to get here, it takes you to maintain here. So when you are feeling all better, you can't leave caution to the wind and go hog wild back into your old ways. You must continue to practise. Now your practice may not need to be as strong or as regimented as it was during your healing phase, but it still need be there. Focus on a consistent practice - because practice does not make perfect, practice makes **progress.**

Meal plans and workout routines?

My friends, food and exercise are an adventure and something that you need to discover for yourself. Food is very intimate and goes inside your body. I could have had a nutritionist or personal trainer design all these fancy recipes and routines, however, you would lose the appreciation for the true essence of food and movement. You must experiment and find what you enjoy and what works best for your body. On the resource page at the back of this book there is a link to purchase the 7 day D-Spot Meal Practice Plan with recipes. This is just to give you some ideas but it truly is best to experiment for yourself by following the guidelines provided in this book.

With food, there is work and love put in to creating meals, and your best bet is to keep ingredients and recipes simple and to your liking.

Explore and be creative with your food. This will create an entirely different dynamic.

But if you feel you require a recipe book, there are many out there that will suit. Look for paleo, and low allergen books.

Please note you will have to make modifications to the ingredients to suit your stage of the D-Spot plan as well as your own personal food sensitivities (another reason I didn't want to include recipes).

With exercise and movement, you will need to find what makes you sing! Vocally sure, but I mean in your heart and soul. Forms of movement or exercise that excite you will help you to stay consistent. Or trust me, you simply will not.

Final notes

The amount of times you repeat this program will depend on your score in the D-Spot quiz, but it should be repeated a minimum of once per year. The Connect and Calm phases should be part of your normal routine, so only the Clean like a Queen phase needs to be repeated. For the most benefit, extend this phase from two weeks to four or six weeks. This is what I do with my patients, and this is the big game changer. Over time you will fall off, and you will be required to reboot your systems. So book it now. Put it in your calendar for next year, where you will re-implement all of these strategies.

If you feel you are still floundering, take a look at my website www. drmarisol.com and follow me on social media to stay connected.

Don't forget you can also contact your local naturopathic doctor and book an appointment to get some guidance as well. This can be life changing and take you where you need to go in life. Look for your country's provincial or state naturopathic association and find a licensed doctor there.

You purchasing this book has already started you on a completely different trajectory than most people who deal with an irritable bowel, irritable bowel disease, or any kind of chronic gut or health ailment.

Life needs to be a balance of effort and ease, or as I like to call it discipline and indulgence. If you indulge all the time you will not be well. If you are disciplined all the time, you miss out on the spontaneity, fun and flavour of life. If you practice a balance of indulging and being disciplined, you will be well. We have seen it with our patients. Those who follow and repeat the plan have huge long term benefits. Those who don't, slip back down into their sick state.

I want to take this time now to really encourage you, and to let you know how proud I am of you for committing to read through this whole book and if you are actively implementing what you have learned. Yes! Do it! I always say, you get out of something what you put into it.

The world really is your oyster, and you can live the legendary life that you want to live.

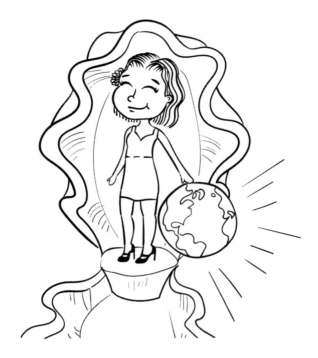

You really can. The first step is learning how to own your throne. Are you owning your throne on a day to day basis? Take the time to make yourself a priority, so that you can be healthy, happy and whole. You can bring to this world your best self!

Do it. Do it now. Do it for you, for your children and for the world. You are here for a reason and you have a unique magic that needs to be brought to light. The only way this will be done, will be with you owning your throne! I bless your journey, and I'm so happy to be part of it with you.

Stay tuned for my upcoming books and programs. Because on this journey of life, we must always keep working so as to evolve into the greatest expression of ourselves, and that takes constant dedication and commitment to education and improvement.

You are worth it. We are worth it. This is what makes life grand!

My ultimate hope with this book and all of my work is to help you find your grace. We all have it. Some of us keep it very hidden, while others wear it on their sleeves. Your gut is interconnected to your grace. What happens on the physical plane is merely a reflection of what is happening in the mental, emotional and spiritual aspects of your life.

All information is provided for educational purposes and is not meant to treat, cure or prevent any disease. It does not construe a patient/doctor relationship. Before undertaking any and all therapies ask your higher power, your gut, and your doctor if it is right for you. We are all unique and individual, and so too should your protocol be. Please talk to your health care partner.

RESOURCES

Color Download of Legends of the Throne
https://drmarisol.com/legends-of-the-throne/

D-Spot Quiz
http://www.drmarisol.com/d-spot-quiz/

50 Shades of Poo Free Download
https://drmarisol.com/50-shades-of-poop/

Food Sensitivity Testing
https://yourlabwork.com/?ref=859

References Download
www.drmarisol.com/oh-shit-references/

Tabata Timer
http://www.tabatatimer.com/

Dirty Dozen and Clean Fifteen Produce Shopping Guides
https://www.ewg.org/

APPENDIX

It is highly recommended to purchase the Queen Kit to supercharge the results of your program. It is a carefully curated collection of Queen of the Thrones™ lifestyle practice products that help you Connect, Clean, Calm and maintain Clarity.

The Queen Kit includes:

- Queen of the Thrones™ heat-less, less-mess, 3-step Castor Oil Pack

- 100% pure, certified organic, cold-pressed, hexane-free, extra virgin Queen of the Thrones™ Castor Oil in an amber glass bottle

- Eau de Throne™ After you Poo Parfum™

- Beauty Sleep Eye Kit with Cosmetic Castor Oil

- Grateful Dung™ Bracelet

ABOUT THE AUTHOR

Dr. Marisol Teijeiro, ND, BA - Queen of the Thrones™ is a world leader renowned for empowering people to improve their digestive and gut health by unlocking secrets found in the number one product our body produces, our stools.

Her life's mission is for the billions of people around the world, both healthy and suffering from digestive issues like constipation, bloating, gas, irritable bowel syndrome, Crohn's disease, ulcerative colitis and more, to understand the inner workings of their bodies.

She's the founder and clinical director of Sanas Health Practice, where she's helped thousands of patients live happy, healthy lives. She teaches at the Canadian College of Naturopathic Medicine, appears as a guest on TV and podcasts, and speaks around the world.

Her passion and first-visit prescription is castor oil and castor oil packs. She shares cutting edge tips and techniques that are scientifically supported, clinically practiced and historically honoured.

INDEX

Coconut 105, 147, 155, 156, 167, 194, 195, 197, 213, 217, 222

Coconut oil 105, 147, 155, 156, 167, 194, 195, 197, 213, 222

Coffee 12, 15, 16, 43, 44, 56, 78, 87, 88, 144, 145, 146, 147, 148, 149, 153, 154, 225, 249, 264

Colitis xi, 3, 299

Conbiotics™ 70, 76, 102, 103, 212, 251

Constipation xi, 1, 2, 15, 24, 98, 100, 178, 247, 251, 299

Copper 238, 239

Coriander 221

Coronary artery disease 213

Crohn's disease 3, 218, 299

Cumin 221

Curcumin 222, 223

Cystic breasts 253

D

Dairy 9, 55, 95, 154, 191, 193, 216, 217, 234

Dairy alternatives 216, 217

Depression 6, 34, 49, 56, 96, 279

Detoxification 63, 64, 176, 202, 221, 222, 223, 224, 225, 226, 232, 238, 267, 268

Diabetes 7, 11, 30, 80, 87, 90, 145, 149

Digestive enzymes 130, 131, 133, 134, 215, 233, 239, 278, 288

Dill 224

Dopamine 6, 9, 46, 56

Dysbiosis 56

E

Eau de Throne™ 60, 77, 127, 223, 255, 256, 297

Endotoxicity 248

Estrogen 86, 107, 176, 177, 227, 255

F

Fasting 6, 110, 142, 143, 144, 145, 147, 149, 150, 154, 155, 156, 157, 158, 167, 171, 173, 213, 248, 286

Fermentation 9, 67, 70, 81, 106, 113, 153, 167, 219, 227

Fish oil 232, 233, 279, 288

Flax seed 167, 205, 206

FODMAP 107, 212

Folic acid 231

Food sensitivities 56, 91, 92, 94, 95, 131, 189, 191, 192, 198, 217, 287, 291

G

GABA 6, 26, 176, 177, 178, 230

Garlic 197, 198, 223, 224

Gastroesophageal reflux disease (GERD) 65, 173, 214, 215, 256

Ginger 167, 224

Glutathione 150, 152, 183, 222, 225, 226, 252, 270

Glycation 223

Glyphosate 84, 86, 234

GMO 84, 85, 157, 210, 233

Grateful Dung™ Bracelet 62, 112, 126, 164, 184, 280, 281, 287, 297

Green tea 43, 88, 106, 116, 118, 144, 145, 147, 148, 149, 150, 151, 152, 153, 155, 156, 162, 164, 215, 216, 224, 225, 248, 249, 264, 267, 271, 278, 288

Gut lining 2, 25, 60, 145, 195, 210, 231, 235, 236

H

HCl 62, 64, 65, 67, 68, 70, 224

Heart disease 7, 114, 207

Premenstrual syndrome (PMS) 56, 252
Probiotic 35, 71, 101, 103, 156, 157,
    164, 175, 231, 233, 234, 235,
    236, 267, 278, 288
Protein powder 167, 171
Psyllium husk 264
Pumpkin seed oil 197, 207

R

Red raspberry tea 227
Reflux 63, 65, 173, 174, 214, 226
Reverse osmosis 228, 265
Rheumatoid arthritis 87, 218
Rice bran 215
Roasting 211
Rooibos 152, 153, 225
Rosemary 77, 127, 223, 255

S

Sarsasparilla 227, 228
Saturated fat 34, 114, 213
Seeds 83, 154, 155, 166, 167, 170, 186,
    187, 197, 204, 205, 206, 207,
    208, 210, 211, 212, 221, 236
Soaking 187, 211, 212, 270
Soy 93, 210
Sprouting 211, 212
Stomach acid 25, 58, 62, 63, 64, 65,
    66, 67, 68, 69, 95, 102, 103, 105,
    126, 133, 134, 156, 163, 224
Sulfur 198, 223, 224

T

Thyroid 178
Tuna 191, 217, 218, 219, 227
Turmeric 92, 222

U

Uterine fibroids 253

V

Vagus nerve 224
Vinegar 95, 188, 203, 215
Vitamin C 214, 235, 268, 269,
    270, 271
Vitamin D 180, 230, 279, 280, 288
Vitamin E 162, 231, 278, 288

W

Wifi 32, 34, 172, 180, 181, 279
Wild game 197, 220

Y

Yogurt 103, 106, 167, 191, 233

Z

Zinc 25, 63, 64, 207, 220, 235, 236